Implementing Culture Change in Long-Term Care

Elaine T. Jurkowski, MSW, PhD, is a professor and Graduate Program Director at Southern Illinois University Carbondale's School of Social Work, where she teaches courses in health and aging policy, research, and program evaluation, and also holds a joint appointment with the Department of Health Education. Dr. Jurkowski's early career experience working in a community public health interdisciplinary setting in Manitoba, Canada as a social worker exposed her to mental health, disability, vocational rehabilitation, and aging programs. These early experiences, coupled with her training in community health sciences and epidemiology, have shaped Dr. Jurkowski's research and practice interests. Dr. Jurkowski has been active within the culture change movement through the Illinois Pioneer Network. She is currently engaged in research to promote the culture change journey in long-term care facilities, and promoting consumer education in changing the culture of long-term care.

Dr. Jurkowski's research has been funded by the National Institutes of Health, The Hartford Foundation, the Health and Human Services Administration, the Administration on Aging, and the Department on Aging, State of Illinois. Her published research articles have focused on the topics of health disparities, access to mental health and health care services, aging, and disability issues. She has held elected offices in the American Public Health Association (APHA), National Association of Social Workers (NASW), the Gerontological Society of America (GSA), and the Illinois Rural Health Association (IRHA). Her work experiences have included consultation within settings in Niger, West Africa; Hong Kong, India, China, Russia, and Egypt. She is the author of *Policy and Program Planning for Older Adults* (2008 Springer Publishing Company), as well as numerous book chapters and professional articles and managing coeditor of *Handbook for Public Health Social Work* (2013, Springer Publishing Company). Dr. Jurkowski's community service includes serving as a member of the board of directors for various not-for-profit health care agencies within the Southern Illinois area. Dr. Jurkowski also serves as an advisor to the Southern Illinois Pioneer Coalition Advisory Board.

Implementing Culture Change in Long-Term Care

Benchmarks and Strategies for Management and Practice

Elaine T. Jurkowski, MSW, PhD

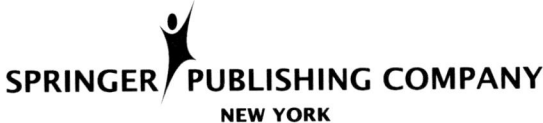

SPRINGER PUBLISHING COMPANY
NEW YORK

Copyright © 2013 Springer Publishing Company, LLC

All rights reserved.

No part of this publication may be reproduced, stored in a retrieval system, or transmitted in any form or by any means, electronic, mechanical, photocopying, recording, or otherwise, without the prior permission of Springer Publishing Company, LLC, or authorization through payment of the appropriate fees to the Copyright Clearance Center, Inc., 222 Rosewood Drive, Danvers, MA 01923, 978-750-8400, fax 978-646-8600, info@copyright.com or on the Web at www.copyright.com.

Springer Publishing Company, LLC
11 West 42nd Street
New York, NY 10036
www.springerpub.com

Acquisitions Editor: Sheri W. Sussman
Production Editor: Joseph Stubenrauch
Composition: diacriTech

ISBN: 978-0-8261-0908-8
e-book ISBN: 978-0-8261-0909-5

13 14 15 / 5 4 3 2 1

The author and the publisher of this Work have made every effort to use sources believed to be reliable to provide information that is accurate and compatible with the standards generally accepted at the time of publication. The author and publisher shall not be liable for any special, consequential, or exemplary damages resulting, in whole or in part, from the readers' use of, or reliance on, the information contained in this book. The publisher has no responsibility for the persistence or accuracy of URLs for external or third-party Internet websites referred to in this publication and does not guarantee that any content on such websites is, or will remain, accurate or appropriate.

Library of Congress Cataloging-in-Publication Data
Implementing culture change in long-term care : benchmarks and strategies for management and practice / Elaine T. Jurkowski.
  p. ; cm.
  Includes bibliographical references and index.
  ISBN 978-0-8261-0908-8 — ISBN 978-0-8261-0909-5 (e-book)
  I. Title.
  [DNLM: 1. Long—Term Care. 2. Benchmarking. 3. Health Services for the Aged. WT 31]
  RA997.A1
  362.16—dc23   2013002643

Special discounts on bulk quantities of our books are available to corporations, professional associations, pharmaceutical companies, health care organizations, and other qualifying groups. If you are interested in a custom book, including chapters from more than one of our titles, we can provide that service as well.

For details, please contact:
Special Sales Department, Springer Publishing Company, LLC
11 West 42nd Street, 15th Floor, New York, NY 10036-8002
Phone: 877-687-7476 or 212-431-4370; Fax: 212-941-7842
E-mail: sales@springerpub.com

Printed in the United States of America by Gasch Printing.

This book is dedicated to my parents, Eddie and Lorraine Jurkowski.

Thank you both for your vision toward "least-restricted environment" as a philosophy toward care for people with mobility limitations and people who are advancing with age.

CONTENTS

Foreword   Bill Thomas, MD   *ix*
Preface   *xiii*
Acknowledgments   *xvii*

PART I—ESTABLISHING A CONTEXT FOR SHAPING LONG-TERM CARE SETTINGS   1

1. The Changing Landscape of Our Long-Term Care Population: The Demographic Shift   3
2. Introduction to Long-Term Care Settings and Culture Change   29
3. Philosophical Paradigms Impacting Long-Term Care Settings   47
4. Artifacts of Culture Change: An Overview of Purpose and Measurement Practices   61

PART II—STRATEGIES AND BENCHMARKS FOR CULTURE CHANGE   85

5. Care Practices   87
6. Environment Benchmarks/Artifacts   111
7. Family and Community Practices   143
8. Leadership Benchmarks/Artifacts   157
9. Workplace Practice Benchmarks/Artifacts   169
10. Outcome Practices   181

PART III—TOOLS AND RESOURCES TO FACILITATE THE CHANGE PROCESS   191

11. The Assessment Process: Identifying a Road Map for Success   193
12. From Assessment to Action: Building on the Planning Process   201
13. Partners for Change: Residents and Family   211

14. Building Coalitions of Effective Change Agent Teams   233

15. Legal and Regulatory Bodies and the Culture Change Process   249

16. A Vision for the Future   261

Appendix A. Resources for Community-Based Agencies and Nonprofit Groups   265

Appendix B. Websites for Culture Change Resources   269

Appendix C. Glossary of Culture Change Vocabulary   271

Bibliography   277

Index   283

FOREWORD

As we begin the journey toward understanding culture change and the role embracing person-centered care, it only seems fitting to share some of my own journey to help illuminate the importance of the turn within the long-term care arena toward the direction of person-centered care.

My own career, which began as an emergency room (ER) physician was drawn to the role of the medical director of a nursing home following a turbulent evening during a 24-hour shift in the ER, responding to a prison fight. Taking on the role of medical director seemed a welcome reprieve for one night per week from the chaos and pace of the ER. The culture of the nursing home was a sharp contrast to the split second decision making and unpredictability of the ER world. Although I quickly fell in love with the nursing home facility's residents, staff, and families, what I had not anticipated was how the experience would transform my life, and the lives of others, as a result of the way my own life was touched and impacted.

My facility, for which I was medical director, was well known for its strict adherence to regulations and the efficiency with which the facility operated. While the facility was deficiency-free and successfully navigated through numerous regulatory and accreditation surveys, for which we boasted a sense of pride, none of us was prepared for the sad reality that residents, although well cared for, did not really feel the care. I was struck by this sobering reality when an old woman whom I had just finished treating with a rash, after treatment, looked me in the eye, and said, "I am so lonely."

Plagues of loneliness, helplessness, and boredom were rampant throughout the facility, despite the fact that the facility offered model medical care to the residents. What became apparent was that as people age, their world gets smaller, and eventually one's world is manifested around them within about 10 feet in diameter. Since we are all a part of this world, we need to ask the question, how do we contribute to the world of each of the residents, and how do we facilitate their world to help them maintain their dignity and person-centeredness and create a world devoid of loneliness, boredom, and helplessness.

The Eden Alternative, an initial step toward battling the plagues of loneliness, boredom, and helplessness was an initial pathway for the long-term care movement to design home environments for frail elderly people. Its philosophy also helped shaped the pioneer network and culture change movement. The importance of elders is one dimension of culture change.

The culture change movement that emerged during the last quarter of the 20th Century was inspired by a profound dissatisfaction with long-term care's status quo. Largely informal in its structure and led by a changing cast of highly energetic advocates, professionals, elders, and family members, the movement has maintained a passion for transforming the language, expectations, and practices that govern how we deliver assistance to older people. It can also be said that, given a choice between advancing theory or practice, advocates for culture change have reliably praised the former and embraced the latter. This bias toward action was also shared by nearly all of America's great 19th Century inventors and most of the movement's leaders would agree with Thomas A. Edison's insistence that "I have not failed, I've just found 10,000 ways that don't work."

This "chewing gum and bailing twine" approach to innovation and change served to inspire the creativity of a leading edge of enthusiastic risk-takers in the field of aging services. It also produced a new vocabulary and design esthetic along with new approaches to the management and structure of organizations providing support to older people. Less happily, this "ad hoc" approach to innovation also hobbled the movement in important but often overlooked ways. At every point along the culture change journey, critics have asked, "Where is the proof?" In fact, there has been precious little with which to answer them. The movement's preference for the empiricism of practice, heavy reliance anecdotes, and the absence of an accessible, carefully crafted consideration of the movement in relation to existing literature has diminished its influence, tarnished its reputation, and slowed progress toward important public policy goals.

The publication of *Implementing Culture Change in Long-Term Care* marks the beginning of a new era in the aging services profession. This book is the Rosetta Stone of the culture change movement. Dr. Jurkowski's skillful blend of theory, research, and practice addresses the movement's most urgent needs and makes the work of culture change advocates accessible to a broader and more influential audience.

Few will be surprised if this work becomes the field's foundational text and remains in print (perhaps in a fifth edition) a quarter century from now. A gifted writer, Dr. Jurkowski's remarkably jargon-free prose easily makes her meaning plain to the reader. Practitioners will find pleasure in being introduced to some of the field's most important theorists and academic audiences will benefit from the introduction she offers to the pragmatic innovations that are already transforming long-term care.

Near the end of her book, Dr. Jurkowski concludes that culture change has, in fact, established itself as an important and enduring element of America's long-term care system. She goes on to ask her readers: "And so, the call is to you. Will you push for strategies that will make a difference in the lives of older people? The challenge lies ahead for each one of us. We are the ambassadors of change." Experience teaches us, as it taught Edison, that such a challenge can rarely be answered by drawing a straight line between a problem (e.g., loneliness) and a solution (a visitation program). In the field of aging services, necessity compels us to connect the technical and cultural dimensions of a problem in creative ways that are both simple and elegant. The value of such a unifying construct can be seen most clearly in the culture change movement's proven ability to craft a new, growth oriented, narrative that can support a solidly developmental approach to aging.

There is a new old age waiting to be born and those who have committed themselves to the culture change movement are destined to be its midwives. This new elderhood is, even now, taking shape in the unlikely environs of America's old age archipelago. To a degree that is much larger than most people realize, the effort to reform long-term care is also capable of transforming the broader cultural understanding of aging. This book offers us a context within which we can consider these changes. It's careful evaluation of the movement's most important strategies, tools, and resources will do much to accelerate change within and beyond the field of long-term care.

This book is the future in paper and ink.

Bill Thomas, MD, Founder of the Eden Alternative
and the Green House Project

PREFACE

The process of change, regardless of the issue or context, is never a simple or singular process. If one were to look at his or her own habits, and how difficult it may be to change something like diet, an exercise regimen, or one's daily routine, it becomes clearer how slow the change process can be. In the world of long-term care settings, a movement has been afoot to change the culture of an entire system, or the "culture" of care. Theoretically or conceptually, this may seem like an easy process; however, because we humans are creatures of habit, and systems have become "institutionalized," the process of culture change in long-term care settings may require a deliberate strategic approach. Consequently, I wrote this book to support administrators and the next generation of long-term care staff to facilitate a culture of dignity and least restrictive environment for residents of long-term care, rehabilitation, and other care settings.

This book is divided into three parts. Part I establishes a context for shaping long-term care settings. Part II explores strategies and benchmarks for culture change, and Part III addresses tools and resources to support the culture change process.

The book begins with an exploration of the changing landscape of our long-term care population. Chapter 1 outlines the landscape of the U.S. aging population and highlights many of the demographic changes we have seen over the last century. These changes are explored as a strategy to predict the need for revised models of long-term care management and practice. The chapter also introduces the context and concepts of the culture change movement.

Chapter 2 examines long-term care settings and explores these settings within the context of culture change. This chapter discusses and describes the various types of long-term care settings available for the provision of care and provides some case examples to help illustrate the typical levels of care and types of services provided. This chapter will be extremely helpful to individuals with limited experience within long-term care settings. It also provides some ideas about how to envision a culture change approach within these settings.

Chapter 3 examines the philosophical paradigms that play a role in the management and operation of long-term care settings. The medical model, rehabilitation/disability paradigm, independent-living, and strengths-based approaches are all compared and contrasted in this chapter, with the end goal of understanding how these practices play a role in long-term care settings. These different models are also explored to help provide readers an understanding of how these paradigms facilitate or impede a culture change model.

Chapter 4 begins to explore a tool developed by the Centers for Medicare & Medicaid Services. The history and development of the Artifacts of Culture Change Tool (ACCT) is reviewed in this chapter. The chapter also examines some of the purpose and measurement practices and empirical principles behind the tool, including its validity and reliability.

Part II explores the ACCT in a broader way, within six specific content areas. It outlines some detailed examples of how these benchmarks have been met through best practice examples and illustrations.

Chapter 5 outlines care practice benchmarks/artifacts. Items/strategies that relate to the actual direct care of people within long-term care settings are explored. Items from the ACCT tool are showcased, with examples from the field given in an effort to provide readers with some ideas as to how to meet the benchmarks. Environment benchmarks/artifacts are explored in Chapter 6, which reviews items/strategies that relate to the environment for people living within long-term care settings. Family and community benchmarks/artifacts are explored in Chapter 7, which also focuses on how to engage the family and community surrounding those living within long-term care settings. Chapter 8 explores leadership benchmarks/artifacts and reviews items/strategies for governance, management, and leadership of long-term care settings. Workplace practice benchmarks/artifacts are outlined in Chapter 9. Within Chapter 9, a review of items/strategies that relate to the culture of the professional care environment within long-term care settings engages readers. Chapter 10 explores outcomes and how to facilitate the best possible outcomes for the purpose of enhancing long-term care settings.

Part III explores tools and resources that will be helpful in facilitating an actual change of culture to meet the benchmarks outlined in Part II. Each chapter in this section provides specific examples for how the skills can be used in the change process to meet some of the benchmarks identified within Part II.

Chapter 11 examines the assessment process and outlines how this process is essential to the identification of a road map for success. Readers will gain a clearer understanding through this chapter of how to use the ACCT in the initial assessment process, where and how to begin, and how to engage stakeholder support both within and outside the facility in efforts to pursue success. The chapter also discusses the needs assessment process and outlines ways to engage in the needs assessment venue for staff within facilities. Chapter 12 builds upon this chapter by moving the assessment process into action, and by expanding on the planning process. The chapter also provides a process to help readers implement strategies to help move benchmarks within facilities through the use of the assessment data obtained in Chapter 11.

I would be remiss if I did not include partners as a vital component of the change process. Chapter 13 addresses how we can integrate two essential components of our team: residents and family. This chapter shares with readers how to engage these partners in the process of culture change through what we know from the scientific literature and examples of best practice. Continuing along the theme of partnerships, the book moves to Chapter 14, which addresses the use of coalitions as effective change agents for team members. This chapter addresses how coalitions (i.e., pioneering coalitions) have been vehicles for change and identifies for readers how to go about building and sustaining such coalitions.

Legal and regulatory agencies also play a critical role in the process of culture change in care facilities. Chapter 15 presents some of the expectations and issues that legal and regulatory entities may impose and that can facilitate or impede the culture change process. The chapter also addresses strategies on how to work with state and federal regulatory bodies, which can be helpful in the process of empowering facility staff to make changes and deal with their surveyors.

The concluding chapter (Chapter 16) summarizes the book, provides an inspirational call to prepare for the future, and attempts to imbue readers with an enthusiasm for the art, craft, and science of culture change.

Appendices A and B contain a series of resources and websites, respectively, that can be used in the process of meeting the specific benchmarks identified. Appendix C provides language which can be used to create a more person-centered environment, and preserve the dignity of the individual.

ACKNOWLEDGMENTS

Any journey, whether it be a building project, running a race, or, in this case, writing a book, never is completed in a vacuum but involves a team of people. This is also true in the case of the completion of this special book. Many people deserve credit for helping me pursue this journey, and if for some reason you are not named individually, please know you are included in my thoughts.

This project would have never come to conception or fruition without the wisdom and vision of Sheri W. Sussman, Executive Editor, Springer Publishing Company. Sheri's initial enthusiasm for a book that would help facilitate the process of culture change sold me on its importance and on the mission I was to embark. Sheri's determination to have the project completed and into the hands of our foot soldiers who would command the mission of culture change helped me see the mission to completion. Katie Corasaniti, Associate Editor at Springer Publishing, was also a tremendous help with the details of production and manuscript development. Joseph Stubenrauch, Production Editor, also provided helpful and insightful guidance through the final production stage.

Numerous people active in the culture change movement have also been an inspiration to me in helping shape the many ideas and directions that this book has taken. Although too numerous to mention, I extend my sincere thanks to you for all that you do to support the lives of people living in long-term care settings. Rindi Reeves, Program Manager at the Egyptian Area Agency on Aging, deserves special mention for her inspiration to pursue the culture change venue. Phil Gillespie, a volunteer and family member, who helped lead the culture change movement in Illinois, deserves special mention for his dedication to the charge and for keeping me abreast of the importance of culture change within long-term care settings. Zoe Dearing, of the Alzheimer's Association of St. Louis, Missouri; Judy Ellet, from the ombudsman's office in Illinois for her vision and commitment; as well as the Illinois Pioneer Coalition Network and the Southern Illinois Pioneer Coalition also deserve thanks. The National Pioneer Coalition Office deserves acknowledgment as well for their help with resources and reports.

The long-term care facilities willing to showcase their innovations deserve acknowledgment. My glimpse into these facilities also merits a special thank you to the many friends and colleagues who made me aware of facilities that we were able to showcase in this book. John Taylor Sr. and Ida Jane Barnard, two residents of rehabilitation and nursing care facilities, who made me keenly aware of the impact of facility practices and environments in this regard, also deserve mention.

My students deserve acknowledgment for their curiosity, questioning, and never-failing vision and commitment to helping reshape the culture of long-term care settings for older adults and people with disabilities. Their vision and questioning have helped me shape the classroom exercises and discussion questions found within this book.

I also would like to thank my student graduate assistants who have helped me throughout the process of working on this book. Early on—Jamie Anderson, Jenn Harvey, and Tim McGrath worked on shaping research initiatives that formed the basis of this book—while Sarah DeWolfe, MSW, helped with the literature searches, tables, editing, and proofreading.

Last, to my dear and loving family, where would this project be without your caring and support, especially from my dear husband Bill? Thank you for your patience, allowing me to be the "absentee wife," and for your hours of editing and proofreading my drafts. The task could never have come to completion without your endless cheerleading and unconditional belief in me.

I

Establishing a Context for Shaping Long-Term Care Settings

The chapters in this first part of the book provide a context for the importance of establishing and moving toward benchmarks in long-term care. They provide an overview of the changing demography that will lead to an increased need for long-term care facilities. The chapters shape one's perspective by framing the different philosophical paradigms that affect continuing and long-term care settings (from the medical model to the strengths-based perspective). This part of the book ends with an overview of the Centers for Medicare & Medicaid Services Artifacts of Culture Change (ACCT) and an outline of its purpose, providing some background to both the instrument and the psychometric properties behind the ACCT tool.

1

The Changing Landscape of Our Long-Term Care Population: The Demographic Shift

If one compares our population today with the demographic makeup of society in 1900, or even in 1950, it is not difficult to recognize the demographic shift that U.S. society has experienced. People today live longer; live independently for a greater period of time; and are expecting to maintain their dignity, autonomy, and ability to direct the world around them through their independent decisions. Social justice movements, which emerged in the early 1960s beginning with the civil rights movement, have moved our social fabric from resignation to activism. These demands have permeated many walks of life, including arenas for people with disabilities and older adults. The end result is a shift in the expectations of our culture, especially as they relate to the care of older adults and/or people with disabilities.

In the United States and Canada, housing for people who are living out their golden years, or for people with disabilities, has historically been institutional or asylum-like and has catered to the most frail and elderly. In years gone by, people who lived in such settings often were without extended or nuclear families to care for their needs. The isolated nature of these individuals led them into care settings that were limited to sterile environments. Since 1997, there has been a movement in the United States to change the culture of nursing homes and assisted living facilities that is based on a belief in person-centered care. Within this model of person-centered care, the values and wishes of residents in care settings are respected and considered. The process of this effort has been characterized as "culture change" or "pioneering," and efforts are underway to attempt to reshape the culture of long-term care.

THE DEMOGRAPHIC SHIFT

Age Breakdown

Older adults have become a growing proportion of the population in the United States and in other countries worldwide. Advances in nutrition, medical technologies, and living conditions have led to the increase in longevity for this segment of the population. In the United States in 2010, more people were age 65 years and older than in any previously documented census period. In addition, there was a rise of 15.1% in the population age 65 and older in 2010 compared with 2000 (Werner, 2011). This is in contrast to other segments of the population, which saw a rise of only 9.7% in its largest growth area between 2000 and 2010.

Over time, there has been a steady increase in the U.S. population base that is age 65 and older. The first published data on population rankings of people age 65 and older, identified in 1870, indicated that this population comprised 1.2 million individuals, or 3% of the total U.S. population. Thirty years later, in 1900, this proportion of the population nearly tripled, to 3.1 million. If we fast forward nearly a century and examine data from the 1990 U.S. Census, we find that 31.2 million people were 65 and older. This figure continued to grow, to 35.0 million in 2000 and 40.3 million in 2010.

Although these numbers showcase a growth in the number of people who are 65 and older, one may argue that the U.S. population in general has also expanded. Thus, this begs the question: What proportion of our population is 65 and older, and how has this proportion of the population grown or changed over time? In the United States in 1900, people who were 65 and older comprised 4.1% of the population (Werner, 2011). This can be sharply contrasted with 1990, when the proportion of people in this age group represented 12.6% of the total population. Between 1990 and 2010, the U.S. Census Bureau reported an increase again in the proportion of this group, to 13.0% of the population. Figure 1.1 provides an overview of the 65-and-older population by size and percentage of the total population between 1900 and 2010.

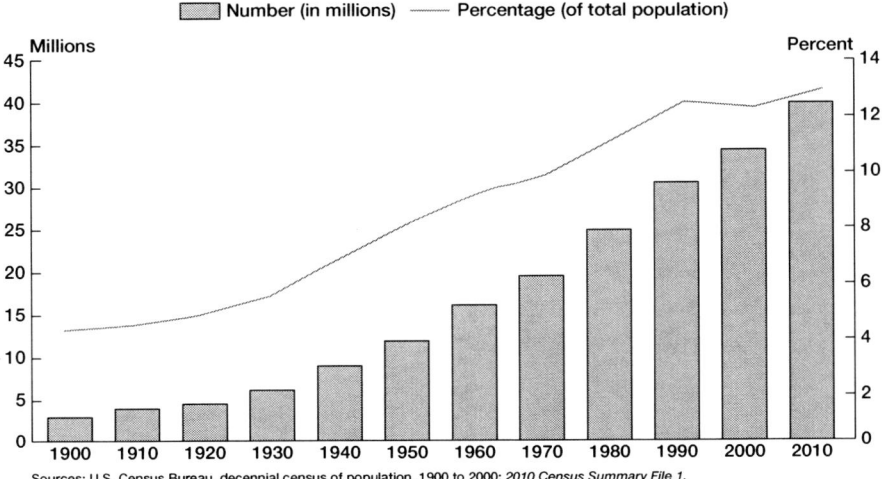

FIGURE 1.1 Population 65 Years and Older: Size and Percentage of the Total Population. Data from the U.S. Census Bureau.

Source: Adapted from Werner (2011).

Thus far we have examined the shifts over time in the general category of people 65 years of age and older. However, the older adult population is generally examined in age segments ranging from 65 to 74 years, 75 to 84 years, 85 to 94 years, and 95+ years. In light of our analysis of the changing demographic landscape, it is also interesting to note how the population has shifted in each of these age segments. Table 1.1 showcases these data and compares each group both in actual number and in percentage change between the year 2000 and the year 2010.

It is noteworthy that the age group that experienced the largest increase between 2000 and 2010 was the 85- to 94-year-old group, which grew from 3.9 million to 5.1 million, or by 29.9%. In addition, individuals age 95 and older demonstrated a strong rate of growth. This group grew from 337,000 (in the year 2000) to 425,000 (in the year 2010), an increase of 25.9%.

Another age group that experienced tremendous growth and change between the year 2000 and the year 2010 is 65- to 69-year-olds, who represent Baby Boomers. This group increased from 9.5 million (in 2000) to 12.4 million (in 2010), an increase of 30.4%. Baby Boomers were born between 1946 and 1964, part of the dramatic increase in birth rates after World War II, and have been categorized as one of the largest generations noted in American history (Hogan, Perez, & Bell, 2008).

Traditionally, women have outnumbered men in the 65 and older population. Although this trend continues, the proportion of men to

TABLE 1.1 Age Breakdown Within Age Groups in the Population 65 Years and Older by Age and Gender: 2000 and 2010

Gender and Age	2000			2010			Change, 2000–2010	
	N	% 65 Years+ Population	% U.S. Total Population	N	% 65 Years+ Population	% U.S. Total Population	N	%
Both sexes, all ages	281,421,906	(X)	100.0	308,745,538	(X)	100.0	27,323,632	9.7
65 years and over	34,991,753	100.0	12.4	40,267,984	100.0	13.0	5,276,231	15.1
65–74 years	18,390,986	52.6	6.5	21,713,429	53.9	7.0	3,322,443	18.1
65–69 years	9,533,545	27.2	3.4	12,435,263	30.9	4.0	2,901,718	30.4
70–74 years	8,857,441	25.3	3.1	9,278,166	23.0	3.0	420,725	4.7
75–84 years	12,361,180	35.3	4.4	13,061,122	32.4	4.2	699,942	5.7
75–79 years	7,415,813	21.2	2.6	7,317,795	18.2	2.4	−98,018	−1.3
80–84 years	4,945,367	14.1	1.8	5,743,327	14.3	1.9	797,960	16.1
85–94 years	3,902,349	11.2	1.4	5,068,825	12.6	1.6	1,166,476	29.9
85–89 years	2,789,818	8.0	1.0	3,620,459	9.0	1.2	830,641	29.8
90–94 years	1,112,531	3.2	0.4	1,448,366	3.6	0.5	335,835	30.2
95 years and over	337,238	1.0	0.1	424,608	1.1	0.1	87,370	25.9
95–99 years	286,784	0.8	0.1	371,244	0.9	0.1	84,460	29.5
100 years and over	50,454	0.1	—	53,364	0.1	—	2,910	5.8

Gender and Age	2000			2010			Change, 2000–2010	
	N	% 65 Years+ Population	% U.S. Total Population	N	% 65 Years+ Population	% U.S. Total Population	N	%
Median age, 65 years and over	74.5	(X)	(X)	74.1	(X)	(X)	−0.4	(X)
Male, all ages	138,053,563	(X)	49.1	151,781,326	(X)	49.2	13,727,763	9.9
65 years and over	14,409,625	41.2	5.1	17,362,960	43.1	5.6	2,953,335	20.5
65–74 years	8,303,274	23.7	3.0	10,096,519	25.1	3.3	1,793,245	21.6
65–69 years	4,400,362	12.6	1.6	5,852,547	14.5	1.9	1,452,185	33.0
70–74 years	3,902,912	11.2	1.4	4,243,972	10.5	1.4	341,060	8.7
75–84 years	4,879,353	13.9	1.7	5,476,762	13.6	1.8	597,409	12.2
75–79 years	3,044,456	8.7	1.1	3,182,388	7.9	1.0	137,932	4.5
80–84 years	1,834,897	5.2	0.7	2,294,374	5.7	0.7	459,477	25.0
85–94 years	1,158,826	3.3	0.4	1,698,254	4.2	0.6	539,428	46.5
85–89 years	876,501	2.5	0.3	1,273,867	3.2	0.4	397,366	45.3
90–94 years	282,325	0.8	0.1	424,387	1.1	0.1	142,062	50.3
95 years and over	68,172	0.2	—	91,425	0.2	—	23,253	34.1
95–99 years	58,115	0.2	—	82,263	0.2	—	24,148	41.6

(continued)

TABLE 1.1 Age Breakdown Within Age Groups in the Population 65 Years and Older by Age and Gender: 2000 and 2010 *(continued)*

Gender and Age	2000			2010			Change, 2000–2010	
	N	% 65 Years+ Population	% U.S. Total Population	N	% 65 Years+ Population	% U.S. Total Population	N	%
100 years and over	10,057	—	—	9,162	—	—	−895	−8.9
Median age, 65 years and over	73.5	(X)	(X)	73.2	(X)	(X)	−0.3	(X)
Female, all ages	143,368,343	(X)	50.9	156,964,212	(X)	50.8	13,595,869	9.5
65 years and over	20,582,128	58.8	7.3	22,905,024	56.9	7.4	2,322,896	11.3
65–74 years	10,087,712	28.8	3.6	11,616,910	28.8	3.8	1,529,198	15.2
65–69 years	5,133,183	14.7	1.8	6,582,716	16.3	2.1	1,449,533	28.2
70–74 years	4,954,529	14.2	1.8	5,034,194	12.5	1.6	79,665	1.6
75–84 years	7,481,827	21.4	2.7	7,584,360	18.8	2.5	102,533	1.4
75–79 years	4,371,357	12.5	1.6	4,135,407	10.3	1.3	−235,950	−5.4
80–84 years	3,110,470	8.9	1.1	3,448,953	8.6	1.1	338,483	10.9
85–94 years	2,743,523	7.8	1.0	3,370,571	8.4	1.1	627,048	22.9

Gender and Age	2000			2010			Change, 2000–2010	
	N	% 65 Years+ Population	% U.S. Total Population	N	% 65 Years+ Population	% U.S. Total Population	N	%
85–89 years	1,913,317	5.5	0.7	2,346,592	5.8	0.8	433,275	22.6
90–94 years	830,206	2.4	0.3	1,023,979	2.5	0.3	193,773	23.3
95 years and over	269,066	0.8	0.1	333,183	0.8	0.1	64,117	23.8
95–99 years	228,669	0.7	0.1	288,981	0.7	0.1	60,312	26.4
100 years and over	40,397	0.1	—	44,202	0.1	—	3,805	9.4
Median age, 65 years and over	75.2	(X)	(X)	74.8	(X)	(X)	−0.4	(X)

Source: U.S. Census Bureau, Census 2000 Summary File 1 and 2010 Census Summary File 1. For information on confidentiality protection, nonsampling error, and definitions, see www.census.gov/prod/cen2010/doc/sf1.pdf.

Note: X = not applicable; dashes indicate that the percentage rounds to 0.0.

women is increasing, and in 2010, there appeared to be a movement toward closing this gender gap. Within the 85- to 94-year-old age range, the number of men increased by 46.5% between 2000 and 2010. Although there was an increase in the proportion of women within this same time period, the increase was only 22.9%. Another age group that showed significant change was 90- to 94-year-old men. Within this age group, the number of men increased by 50.3% from 2000 to 2010. In contrast, women within this same age group grew by only 23.3%.

The number of centenarians (people over 100 years of age) has also increased over time, and currently the United States has more than ever reported in history. Within this category, the 2010 census still indicates a gender gap: The number of women in this category grew by 9.4%, but the number of men declined 8.9%.

This change in the demographic landscape of people age 65 and older suggests the importance that housing options will play for this segment of the population in the future, especially within the groups of the oldest-old (85+). However, it is also important to examine what other factors will play a role in defining housing option needs while looking at variables such as marital status, mobility status, health status, and housing tenure.

Marital Status

Marital status is usually an indicator of social support for people, especially as they grow older. Married couples seem to be most prevalent among the young-old (65–74 years), but their numbers decline with age and widowhood increases as we move across the life span of people age 65 and older. The 2010 U.S. Census revealed that 64.7% of couples remained married in the 65- to 74-year-old age group, as compared with 51.7% in the 75- to 84-year-old age group and 31.5% in the 85+ group. In contrast, widowhood almost quadrupled for those in the 85+ age group (59.6%) as compared with people in the 65-to-74 age range (15.8% widowed). An interesting observation is that people within the oldest-old category appear to be more stable in their relationships. Only 4.4% of those in the 85+ years category reported being divorced in 2010, as compared with 16.5% of people in the 55- to 59-year-old group. In contrast, 13.1% of people in the 65-to-74 category reported being divorced, as compared with 7.1% within the 75-to-84 age range (U.S. Census Bureau, 2010). These figures and other comparisons on marital status can be found in Table 1.2 and are illustrated in Figure 1.2.

The gender differences reflected in the category of marital status are very significant, with women in all age groups more likely to be living

TABLE 1.2 Marital Status of the Age 65 and Over Population, by Age Group and Gender, 2010

Gender and Marital Status	65 +		65–74		75–84		85 +	
Both sexes	%	SE	%	SE	%	SE	%	SE
Total	100.0	0.0	100.0	0.0	100.0	0.0	100.0	0.0
Married[a]	57.6	0.4	66.2	0.5	52.8	0.7	32.0	1.1
Widowed	28.1	0.4	15.8	0.4	36.5	0.7	59.6	1.2
Divorced	10.0	0.2	13.1	0.4	7.1	0.4	4.4	0.5
Never married	4.3	0.2	4.9	0.2	3.6	0.3	4.0	0.5
Men								
Total	100.0	0.0	100.0	0.0	100.0	0.0	100.0	0.0
Married[a]	74.5	0.5	78.0	0.7	73.2	1.0	58.3	2.0
Widowed	12.7	0.4	6.4	0.4	17.2	0.8	34.6	1.9
Divorced	8.7	0.4	11.0	0.5	6.1	0.5	3.9	0.8
Never married	4.1	0.2	4.5	0.3	3.5	0.4	3.2	0.7
Women								
Total	100.0	0.0	100.0	0.0	100.0	0.0	100.0	0.0
Married[a]	44.5	0.5	55.9	0.8	38.1	0.9	18.0	1.1
Widowed	39.9	0.5	24.0	0.7	50.4	0.9	72.9	1.3
Divorced	11.1	0.3	15.0	0.5	7.9	0.5	4.7	0.6
Never married	4.5	0.2	5.1	0.3	3.6	0.3	4.5	0.6

Source: U.S. Census Bureau, Current Population Survey, Annual Social and Economic Supplement, 2010.
Note: These data refer to the civilian noninstitutionalized population.
[a]Includes married, spouse present; married, spouse absent; and separated.

without a spouse or to be widowed. Men in the 65-to-74 age category are reported to be married with a spouse in 75.2% of the age group, as compared with 53.7% among the women in the same age category. This is in contrast to the oldest-old group, in which 55.7% of men reported being married with a spouse as compared with only 16.3% of women reporting this. In this same group of people age 85 and older, 72.9% of women reported having been widowed, compared with only 34.6% of men. In the 65-to-74 group, only 6.4% of men reported being widowed, compared with 23.9% of women in the same age range, during the 2010 census (U.S. Census Bureau, 2010).

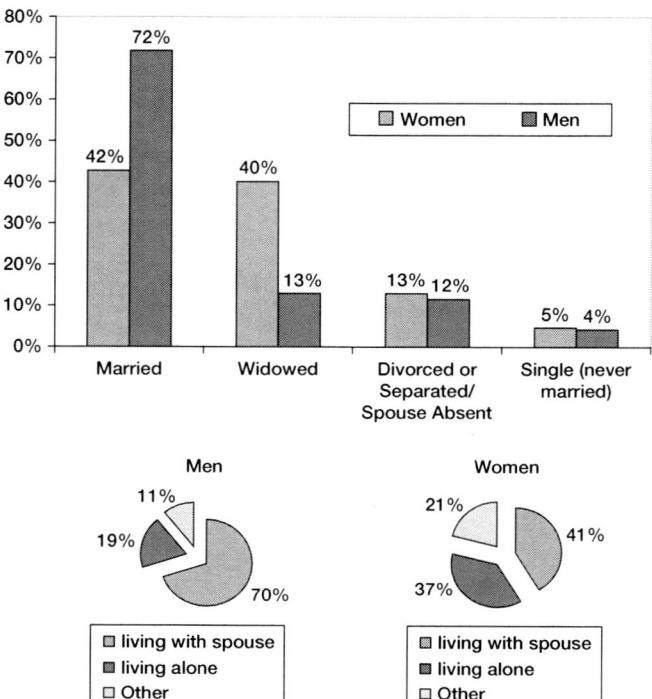

FIGURE 1.2 Marital Status of Persons Age 65 and Older, 2010
Source: U.S. Bureau of the Census (2010).

These stark differences suggest some interesting dynamics when considering marital status within the demographic profile. Because women are generally in the role of caregiver, men will most likely receive care within their natural setting/home, from their spouse, across age groups. Women, however, may be in need of care if they outlive their spouses. This dynamic has implications for long-term care settings that take into account gender differences and individuals' preferences within their environment and care settings.

Mobility Status

Table 1.3 provides an overview of the overall population and racial breakdown of people across age groups who remain in their homes and home-based communities, or who move, either within the county or out of state. Across all age groups these figures appear fairly stable, suggesting that people want to remain within their own home and community.

TABLE 1.3 Mobility Status of the Population 55 Years and Over by Gender and Age: 2009–2010

Gender and Mobility Status	Total 55 Years and Over		55–59 Years		60–64 Years		65–74 Years		75–84 Years		85 Years and Over		65 Years and Over	
	Number	%	Number	%	Number	%	Number	%	Number	%	Number	%	Number	%
Both sexes	74,008	100.0	19,172	100.0	16,223	100.0	20,956	100.0	12,964	100.0	4,693	100.0	38,613	100.0
Nonmover	70,702	95.5	18,106	94.4	15,405	95.0	20,081	95.8	12,586	97.1	4,523	96.4	37,191	96.3
Mover[a]	3,306	4.5	1,066	5.6	818	5.0	875	4.2	378	2.9	170	3.6	1,422	3.7
Same state	2,756	3.7	903	4.7	683	4.2	710	3.4	325	2.5	135	2.9	1,171	3.0
Same county	2,056	2.8	673	3.5	509	3.1	520	2.5	246	1.9	107	2.3	873	2.3
Different county	701	0.9	230	1.2	174	1.1	190	0.9	79	0.6	28	0.6	297	0.8
Different state	486	0.7	145	0.8	118	0.7	149	0.7	43	0.3	31	0.7	223	0.6
Abroad	64	0.1	18	0.1	17	0.1	16	0.1	9	0.1	3	0.1	28	0.1
Male	33,778	100.0	9,318	100.0	7,667	100.0	9,735	100.0	5,427	100.0	1,631	100.0	16,793	100.0
Nonmover	32,213	95.4	8,799	94.4	7,255	94.6	9,309	95.6	5,283	97.3	1,567	96.1	16,159	96.2
Mover[a]	1,564	4.6	518	5.6	412	5.4	426	4.4	144	2.7	64	3.9	634	3.8
Same state	1,312	3.9	444	4.8	355	4.6	338	3.5	128	2.4	48	2.9	513	3.1
Same county	990	2.9	337	3.6	264	3.4	246	2.5	107	2.0	38	2.3	390	2.3

(continued)

TABLE 1.3 Mobility Status of the Population 55 Years and Over by Gender and Age: 2009–2010 (continued)

Gender and Mobility Status	Total 55 Years and Over		55–59 Years		60–64 Years		65–74 Years		75–84 Years		85 Years and Over		65 Years and Over	
	Number	%	Number	%	Number	%	Number	%	Number	%	Number	%	Number	%
Different county	321	1.0	107	1.1	91	1.2	92	0.9	21	0.4	10	0.6	123	0.7
Different state	228	0.7	70	0.8	50	0.7	80	0.8	16	0.3	13	0.8	108	0.6
Abroad	24	0.1	5	0.1	7	0.1	9	0.1	1	-	3	0.2	13	0.1
Female	40,230	100.0	9,854	100.0	8,556	100.0	11,221	100.0	7,537	100.0	3,062	100.0	21,820	100.0
Nonmover	38,489	95.7	9,307	94.4	8,149	95.2	10,773	96.0	7,303	96.9	2,957	96.6	21,032	96.4
Mover[a]	1,742	4.3	547	5.6	406	4.8	449	4.0	234	3.1	106	3.4	788	3.6
Same state	1,444	3.6	459	4.7	328	3.8	372	3.3	198	2.6	87	2.9	657	3.0
Same county	1,065	2.6	336	3.4	246	2.9	274	2.4	140	1.9	70	2.3	483	2.2
Different county	379	0.9	123	1.2	82	1.0	98	0.9	58	0.8	18	0.6	174	0.8
Different state	258	0.6	75	0.8	68	0.8	70	0.6	27	0.4	18	0.6	115	0.5
Abroad	40	0.1	14	0.1	11	0.1	7	0.1	9	0.1	—	—	16	0.1

Source: U.S. Census Bureau, Current Population Survey, Annual Social and Economic Supplement, 2010.
Note: Numbers are in thousands and represent the civilian noninstitutionalized population, plus members of the armed forces living on post or with their families on post.
[a] People who lived in a different home in 2010 than they did in 2009.

Health Status

One's health status plays a critical role in the ability to function and enjoy quality of life. Earlier in this chapter, data were presented that suggested that older adults are living longer than they did a century ago. Despite this shift in mortality and life span, how do older adults perceive their overall health status? Data from the National Center for Health Statistics (2010) reveal that, between the years 2000 and 2009, 40.0% of noninstitutionalized older persons identified their perceived health as excellent or very good (compared with 64.7% for all persons age 18–64 years). Both men and women reported these perceptions, with little differences in the percentages. However, racial differences in perceived health status were evident. African Americans (26.0%), American Indians/Alaska Natives (24.3%), and older Hispanics (28.2%) were less likely to rate their health as excellent or very good compared with Caucasians (42.8%) or Asians (35.3%). Figure 1.3 illustrates these data. The majority of older people have at least one chronic condition, and many have multiple conditions. In 2007–2009, the most frequent health issues reported by people age 65 and older included uncontrolled hypertension (34%), diagnosed arthritis (50%), all types of heart disease (32%), any cancer (23%), diabetes (19%), and sinusitis (14%). Figure 1.4 showcases this data.

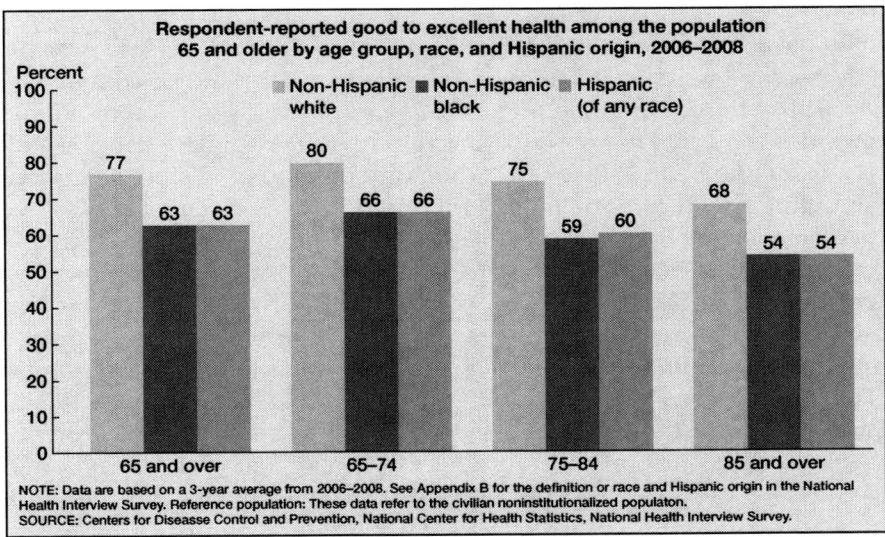

FIGURE 1.3 Perceived Health Status by Ethnicity

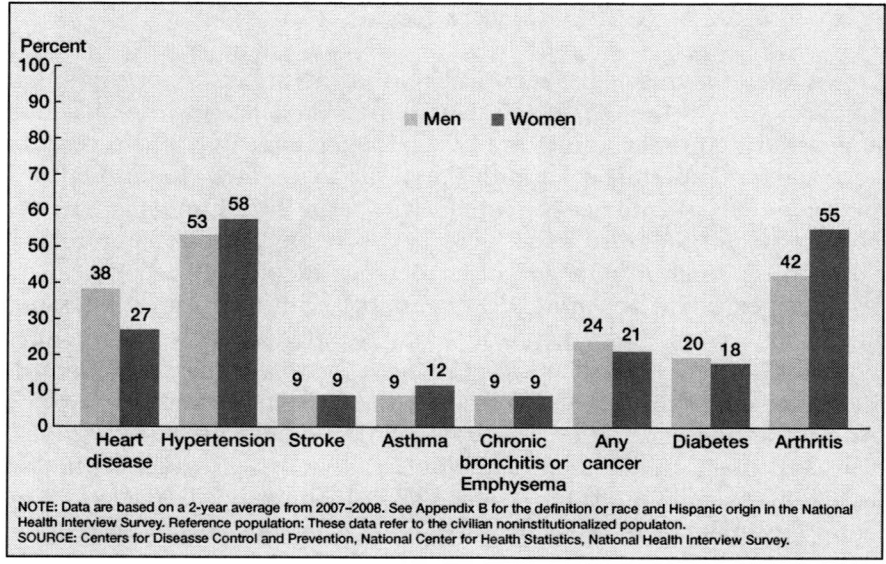

FIGURE 1.4 Chronic Health Conditions Reported by People Age 65 and Older

Almost 63% of people over age 65 reported in 2010 that they had received an influenza vaccination during the past 12 months, and 59% of this same group reported that they had received a pneumococcal vaccination at least once during their lifetime. Almost 35% of people in the 65-to-74 age group, and 24% of people age 75 and older, reported that they participated in some form of regular leisure time physical activity. Of people 65 years and older in the sample, only 9.5% indicated that they smoked at the current time, and only 5% of this same group reported that they drank alcohol to excess (National Center for Health Statistics, 2010).

Some type of disability (i.e., difficulty in hearing, vision, cognition, ambulation, self-care, or independent living) was reported by 37% of people over age 65 in 2010. Some of these disabilities may be relatively minor, but others cause people to require assistance to meet important personal needs. Reported disability increases with age: Fifty-six percent of people over age 80 reported a severe disability, and 29% of people over age 80 reported that they needed some sort of physical assistance. There is a relationship between disability status and reported health status. Among those age 65+ with a severe disability, 64% reported their health as fair or poor. Among the people age 65+ who reported no disability, only 10% reported their health as fair or poor. Presence of a severe disability is also associated with lower annual income and lower levels of education (Federal Interagency Forum on Aging-Related Statistics, 2010).

In terms of the ability to perform specific activities of daily living (ADL), over 27% of community-resident Medicare beneficiaries over age 65 in 2009 had difficulty performing one or more ADL, and an additional 12.7% reported difficulties with instrumental activities of daily living (IADL; Federal Interagency Forum on Aging-Related Statistics, 2010). These ADL included bathing, feeding, going to the bathroom, transferring from bed to chair/wheelchair, getting around in one's home, and dressing oneself. IADL included shopping, using the telephone, conducting banking transactions, managing finances, doing housework, taking medications, and preparing meals. By contrast, 95% of people residing in long-term care settings who were receiving Medicare benefits had difficulties with one or more ADL, and 74% of them had difficulty with three or more ADL (Federal Interagency Forum on Aging-Related Statistics, 2010). The presence of chronic health conditions increases with age, and such conditions affect one's ability to carry out daily activities. As shown in Figure 1.5, the rate of limitations in activities among people in the 85+ group is much higher than that for people in the 65-to-74 age groups.

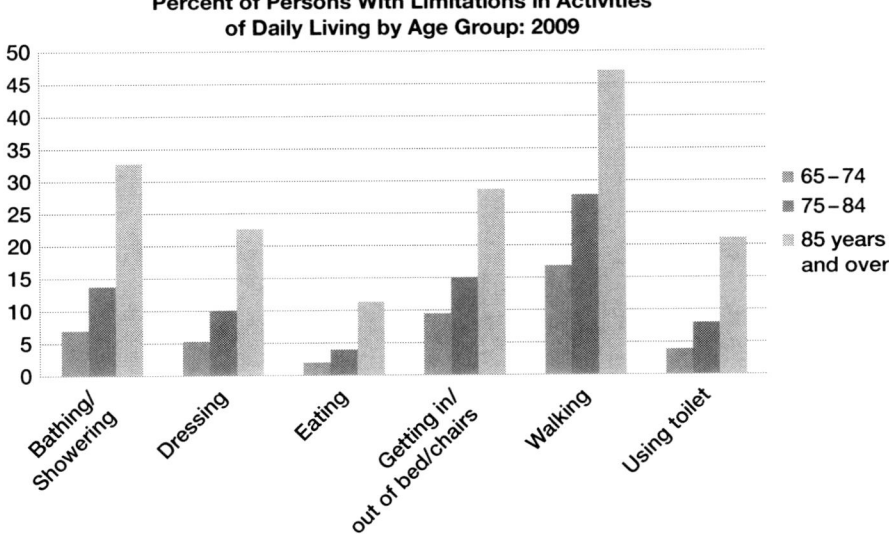

FIGURE 1.5 Activity/Mobility Status by Age Group: 2009

Source: Americans with Disabilities: 2005, December 2008, P70–117 and other Internet releases of data from the U.S. Census Bureau, the Centers for Medicare & Medicaid, and the National Center for Health Statistics, including the National Center for Health Statistics Health Data Interactive Data Warehouse (Administration on Aging, p.15). http://www.aoa.gov/aoaroot/aging_statistics/Profile/2011/docs/2011profile.pdf

Housing for People 55+

Most people perceive their housing as their haven. Owner-occupied housing is critically important for the majority of people within North American society. The "American Dream" was characterized by people working to attain property and assets, especially immigrants. Interestingly, an examination of owner-occupied housing across age groups reveals a trend among married people toward renting as opposed to owning, as one moves across age groups, at least according to the 2010 census. Whereas 92.6% of the population age 65 to 74 owned their residences (U.S. Census, 2010), 90.9% of the 75-to-84 age group owned and occupied their home compared with 86% in the 85+ group. In contrast, women were more likely to own and occupy their home in the 85+ age group (90.4%), compared with only a 77.1% rate of owner-occupied housing in the 65-to-74 age category. Men were more likely to own and occupy their home in the older age range categories. For example, men in the 65-to-74 age category represent 75.7% of men in this older age group residing in their own residence, as compared with 86.7% residing in owner-occupied homes within the 75-to-84 age group, and 85.2% of men owned and occupied their dwelling in the 85+ group. Table 1.4 presents these data in a more comprehensive way.

These data suggest that independence and ownership, as well as autonomy, remain important to people especially as they age. There is a notion that a large proportion of people transfer property to children at a certain age in an effort to hide assets and in preparation for using state-based Medicaid programs for long-term care. Despite the perception that financial planning for long term care, and asset transfer is critical, older adults do want to, and are remaining in their own homes. This fallacy of asset transfer, however does not bear out according to the U.S. 2010 Census. People want to remain as independent as possible. Thus, if long-term care does become a necessity for an older adult, they still want to maintain as much independence and control over their lives and their environment as possible.

Housing Tenure

The term *housing tenure* refers to the people with whom one lives, be they family or nonfamily, and the type of setting or domicile one inhabits. According to the 2010 U.S. Census, in all age groups, seniors who lived with family were also more likely to live in owner-occupied homes. People in the 65-to-74 age group who lived with family reported living in owner-occupied homes in 90.2% of cases, as compared with 68.8% of individuals in the same age group who lived in owner-occupied homes with nonfamily. Across age groups, there appears to be

TABLE 1.4 Housing Tenure by Family Type and Age of Householder 55 Years and Over: 2010

Family Type and Tenure[b]	Total N	Total %	55–59 Years N	55–59 Years %	60–64 Years N	60–64 Years %	65–74 Years N	65–74 Years %	75–84 Years N	75–84 Years %	85 Years and Over N	85 Years and Over %	65 Years and Over N	65 Years and Over %
Family households[c]	27,103	100.0	7,445	100.0	6,262	100.0	8,066	100.0	4,224	100.0	1,106	100.0	13,397	100.0
Owner occupied	23,953	88.4	6,388	85.8	5,535	88.4	7,274	90.2	3,792	89.8	964	87.1	12,030	89.8
Renter occupied	3,150	11.6	1,057	14.2	726	11.6	792	9.8	432	10.2	142	12.9	1,367	10.2
Married-couple families	22,290	100.0	6,093	100.0	5,312	100.0	6,835	100.0	3,308	100.0	742	100.0	10,885	100.0
Owner occupied	20,330	91.2	5,506	90.4	4,851	91.3	6,329	92.6	3,006	90.9	638	86.0	9,972	91.6
Renter occupied	1,960	8.8	587	9.6	460	8.7	506	7.4	303	9.1	104	14.0	913	8.4
Male householder[d]	1,125	100.0	359	100.0	270	100.0	237	100.0	197	100.0	62	100.0	496	100.0
Owner occupied	878	78.1	271	75.4	205	75.9	179	75.7	170	86.7	53	85.2	403	81.2
Renter occupied	246	21.9	88	24.6	65	24.1	58	24.3	26	13.3	9	14.8	93	18.8
Female householder[d]	3,688	100.0	993	100.0	680	100.0	994	100.0	719	100.0	302	100.0	2,016	100.0
Owner occupied	2,745	74.4	611	61.6	479	70.4	766	77.1	616	85.6	273	90.4	1,655	82.1
Renter occupied	943	25.6	381	38.4	201	29.6	228	22.9	104	14.4	29	9.6	361	17.9

Source: U.S. Census Bureau, Current Population Survey, Annual Social and Economic Supplement, 2010.
Note: Numbers are in thousands and represent the civilian noninstitutionalized population, plus members of the armed forces living off post or with their families on post.
[a] Renter households include occupiers who paid no cash in rent.
[b] Households in which at least one member is relationed to the person who owns or rents the occupied housing unit (householder).
[c] No spouse present.

no trend in owner-occupied residential settings, either higher or lower. For example, 68% of people in the 85+ age group reported living in owner-occupied settings with nonfamily, compared with 68.8% of individuals in the 65-to-74 group. Across all age groups, however, it appears that seniors living with family were more likely to reside in owner-occupied settings, whereas people living with nonfamily were more likely to be in renter-occupied settings, in at least one third of cases. Table 1.5 outlines these data from the 2010 U.S. Census.

Education

Education plays an important role in one's preferences and expectations about one's health and well-being. A closer review of data from the 2010 U.S. Census on educational attainment reveals that there is a trend toward higher education in the young-old (65–74 years) when compared with the oldest age group, people 85+ years. The group of people 85+ years of age with less than a bachelor's degree was reported to be 86.9% as compared with 78.5% in the age group of people 65 to 74 years of age. This is in stark contrast to the group of people age 55 to 59 years with 70.3% of people within this age category having less than a bachelor's degree. In addition, the oldest age group (85+) had the highest percentage of individuals with less than a high school degree (26.8%) as compared to 16.7% who reported that they had less than a high school education in the 65-to-74 age group (U.S. Census Bureau, 2010). These data, along with a more comprehensive overview of educational attainment, are illustrated in Table 1.6.

Thus far, we have examined a series of data to showcase some of the trends across the various age cohorts within the U.S. aging population. Although trying to digest these trends may seem an arduous task, they are important in that they paint a picture of the cohort differences across the various age groups within our aging population. Areas such as population density, morbidity, health conditions, housing preferences, and education will all play a role in the expectations for care and housing as people grow older and require either in-home supports or institutional settings.

IMPLICATIONS FOR LONG-TERM CARE AND COMMUNITY PRACTICE SETTINGS

The changing landscape of aging cohorts will have some serious implications for long-term and community care practice settings over the next few decades to come (Jurkowski, 2008). As more baby boomers retire, we can project these changes to roll out in 2015. People today are living longer and remaining in the community within

TABLE 1.5 Housing Tenure by Household Type and Age of Householder 55 Years and Over: 2010

Household Type and Tenure[a]	Total 55 Years and Over N	%	55–59 Years N	%	60–64 Years N	%	65–74 Years N	%	75–84 Years N	%	85 Years and Over N	%	65 Years and Over N	%
Total households	45,658	100.0	10,723	100.0	9,665	100.0	13,164	100.0	8,733	100.0	3,374	100.0	25,270	100.0
Owner occupied	36,494	79.9	8,389	78.2	7,738	80.1	10,782	81.9	7,079	81.1	2,506	74.3	20,367	80.6
Renter occupied	9,163	20.1	2,334	21.8	1,927	19.9	2,382	18.1	1,654	18.9	867	25.7	4,903	19.4
Family households[b]	27,103	100.0	7,445	100.0	6,262	100.0	8,066	100.0	4,224	100.0	1,106	100.0	13,397	100.0
Owner occupied	23,953	88.4	6,388	85.8	5,535	88.4	7,274	90.2	3,792	89.8	964	87.1	12,030	89.8
Renter occupied	3,150	11.6	1,057	14.2	726	11.6	792	9.8	432	10.2	142	12.9	1,367	10.2
Nonfamily households	18,555	100.0	3,278	100.0	3,403	100.0	5,098	100.0	4,508	100.0	2,268	100.0	11,874	100.0
Owner occupied	12,541	67.6	2,001	61.0	2,203	64.7	3,507	68.8	3,287	72.9	1,542	68.0	8,337	70.2
Renter occupied	6,014	32.4	1,277	39.0	1,200	35.3	1,590	31.2	1,221	27.1	725	32.0	3,537	29.8

Source: U.S. Census Bureau, Current Population Survey, Annual Social and Economic Supplement, 2010.

Note: Numbers are in thousands and represent the civilian noninstitutionalized population, plus members of the armed forces living off post or with their families on post.

[a] Renter households include occupiers who paid no cash in rent.

[b] Households in which at least one member is relationed to the person who owns or rents the occupied housing unit (householder).

TABLE 1.6 Educational Attainment of the Population 55 Years and Over by Gender and Age: 2010

Gender and Educational Attainment	Total 55 Years and Over		55–59 Years		60–64 Years		65–74 Years		75–84 Years		85 Years and Over		65 Years and Over	
	N	%	N	%	N	%	N	%	N	%	N	%	N	%
Both sexes	74,008	100.0	19,172	100.0	16,223	100.0	20,956	100.0	12,964	100.0	4,693	100.0	38,613	100.0
Less than 9th grade	5,558	7.5	825	4.3	809	5.0	1,636	7.8	1,551	12.0	738	15.7	3,925	10.2
9th to 12th grade (no diploma)	6,051	8.2	1,155	6.0	904	5.6	1,935	9.2	1,528	11.8	529	11.3	3,992	10.3
High school graduate	25,125	33.9	5,979	31.2	5,089	31.4	7,418	35.4	4,909	37.9	1,730	36.9	14,057	36.4
Some college or associate's degree	17,354	23.4	5,343	27.9	4,062	25.0	4,670	22.3	2,393	18.5	886	18.9	7,949	20.6
Bachelor's degree	11,659	15.8	3,565	18.6	3,028	18.7	2,964	14.1	1,557	12.0	545	11.6	5,066	13.1
Advanced degree	8,261	11.2	2,305	12.0	2,331	14.4	2,335	11.1	1,025	7.9	265	5.6	3,625	9.4
Less than high school graduate	11,609	15.7	1,980	10.3	1,713	10.6	3,571	17.0	3,079	23.8	1,267	27.0	7,917	20.5
High school graduate or more	62,399	84.3	17,193	89.7	14,510	89.4	17,386	83.0	9,885	76.2	3,425	73.0	30,696	79.5
Less than bachelor's degree	54,088	73.1	13,302	69.4	10,864	67.0	15,658	74.7	10,382	80.1	3,883	82.7	29,923	77.5
Bachelor's degree or more	19,920	26.9	5,871	30.6	5,359	33.0	5,298	25.3	2,582	19.9	810	17.3	8,691	22.5
Male	33,778	100.0	9,318	100.0	7,667	100.0	9,735	100.0	5,427	100.0	1,631	100.0	16,793	100.0

	Total 55 Years and Over		55–59 Years		60–64 Years		65–74 Years		75–84 Years		85 Years and Over		65 Years and Over	
	N	%	N	%	N	%	N	%	N	%	N	%	N	%
Less than 9th grade	2,570	7.6	441	4.7	415	5.4	774	8.0	689	12.7	251	15.4	1,714	10.2
9th to 12th grade (no diploma)	2,611	7.7	548	5.9	435	5.7	847	8.7	595	11.0	186	11.4	1,628	9.7
High school graduate	10,399	30.8	2,890	31.0	2,140	27.9	3,145	32.3	1,722	31.7	502	30.8	5,370	32.0
Some college or associate's degree	7,672	22.7	2,496	26.8	1,861	24.3	2,085	21.4	950	17.5	282	17.3	3,316	19.7
Bachelor's degree	6,013	17.8	1,758	18.9	1,657	21.6	1,525	15.7	805	14.8	269	16.5	2,598	15.5
Advanced degree	4,512	13.4	1,185	12.7	1,160	15.1	1,360	14.0	667	12.3	141	8.6	2,167	12.9
Less than high school graduate	5,181	15.3	989	10.6	850	11.1	1,621	16.7	1,284	23.7	437	26.8	3,342	19.9
High school graduate or more	28,597	84.7	8,329	89.4	6,817	88.9	8,114	83.3	4,144	76.3	1,194	73.2	13,451	80.1
Less than bachelor's degree	23,253	68.8	6,375	68.4	4,850	63.3	6,851	70.4	3,956	72.9	1,221	74.9	12,027	71.6
Bachelor's degree or more	10,525	31.2	2,943	31.6	2,816	36.7	2,884	29.6	1,472	27.1	410	25.1	4,766	28.4
Female	40,230	100.0	9,854	100.0	8,556	100.0	11,221	100.0	7,537	100.0	3,062	100.0	21,820	100.0
Less than 9th grade	2,988	7.4	383	3.9	394	4.6	862	7.7	862	11.4	487	15.9	2,211	10.1

(continued)

TABLE 1.6 Educational Attainment of the Population 55 Years and Over by Gender and Age: 2010 *(continued)*

	Total 55 Years and Over		55–59 Years		60–64 Years		65–74 Years		75–84 Years		85 Years and Over		65 Years and Over	
	N	%	N	%	N	%	N	%	N	%	N	%	N	%
9th to 12th grade (no diploma)	3,440	8.6	607	6.2	469	5.5	1,088	9.7	933	12.4	344	11.2	2,365	10.8
High school graduate	14,725	36.6	3,089	31.3	2,949	34.5	4,273	38.1	3,187	42.3	1,228	40.1	8,687	39.8
Some college or associate's degree	9,682	24.1	2,847	28.9	2,201	25.7	2,585	23.0	1,443	19.2	604	19.7	4,633	21.2
Bachelor's degree	5,646	14.0	1,808	18.3	1,371	16.0	1,439	12.8	753	10.0	275	9.0	2,467	11.3
Advanced degree	3,749	9.3	1,120	11.4	1,172	13.7	975	8.7	358	4.7	125	4.1	1,458	6.7
Less than high school graduate	6,429	16.0	990	10.0	863	10.1	1,949	17.4	1,796	23.8	831	27.1	4,575	21.0
High school graduate or more	33,802	84.0	8,864	90.0	7,693	89.9	9,272	82.6	5,741	76.2	2,232	72.9	17,245	79.0
Less than bachelor's degree	30,835	76.6	6,927	70.3	6,013	70.3	8,807	78.5	6,426	85.3	2,662	86.9	17,895	82.0
Bachelor's degree or more	9,395	23.4	2,928	29.7	2,543	29.7	2,414	21.5	1,111	14.7	400	13.1	3,925	18.0

Source: U.S. Census Bureau, Current Population Survey, Annual Social and Economic Supplement, 2010.
Note: Numbers are in thousands and represent the civilian noninstitutionalized population, plus members of the armed forces living off post or with their families on post.

noninstitutionalized settings longer than at any other point of time in history. As people in the younger cohorts (the 65-to-74 age group) become older, or as they become caregivers and advocates for their aging parents (the 85+ age group), their expectations will be different than those currently considered frail elderly. This younger cohort is better educated than their older counterparts, more likely to live alone or with nonfamily, and more likely to not have been married their entire adult life. This younger cohort is also healthier than their older cohort peers and has more mobility in terms of ADL and IADL. Regardless of the cohort, people appear to want to remain in their own homes and community settings, and tend not to be actively mobile in terms of change of residence. The implications of some of these demographic trends will include the fact that people who will eventually reside in long-term care settings will be less physically mobile, have more chronic health conditions, and probably will also be more frail. Education equips people with the ability to exercise more control over themselves and their environment. Inherent within this control is the expectation that one's personal attributes, wishes, and values will be recognized, valued, and respected by those around one. This group also expects that encounters with helping professionals will be relationship oriented and include their own voice in decisions made about their personhood.

This value and belief system will not cease once a person needs assistance with his or her care needs and regimens. In fact, it may actually become more pronounced with time and age. Thus, the importance of reframing our current long-term care delivery system becomes of paramount importance.

According to Kapp (2012), the restrictive, regimented culture of nursing homes and long-term care settings is beginning to change and move toward homelike, welcoming environments. The focus in these environments should be on close interpersonal relationships between residents and staff who are empowered to respond to the residents' needs, values, and personal preferences. The demographic changes that will abound in the future will help push the issue of person-centered environments within care settings to the forefront.

CULTURE CHANGE AS A SOLUTION

The concept of person-centered care settings has been embraced by a movement identified as *culture change*, which first originated in the United States following a summit in Washington, DC, in 2003. The Eden Alternative movement, which preceded the culture change movement, paved the way for person-centered environments and settings.

Proponents of culture change hope to pave the way for a renewed set of benchmarks within long-term care settings. The philosophy of the culture change movement has occurred simultaneously with changes in the disability movement recognized over the past few decades, as well as with the concept of "normalization" (Wolfensberger, 1972, 1980). The culture change movement values the importance of individualized care and personal desires and is based on the principles of community, affiliation, and belonging. Schoeneman and Bowman (2006) developed an instrument to help facilitate these philosophical changes. The instrument referred to as "Artifacts for Culture Change" incorporates the philosophy of person-first and individualized values.

This book is designed to help readers understand and facilitate changes to long-term care settings and to meet the challenges that this shift in paradigm will present. Each of the three parts of this book is designed to help equip readers with tools and strategies to effect change. Although, as mentioned in the Preface, systemwide changes in habits, systems, or environments may seem daunting or even impossible, the first step is to visualize and believe that such change is indeed possible. This vision and commitment are the key ingredients for influencing the culture of long-term care settings.

DISCUSSION/REFLECTION QUESTIONS

1. *Describe some of the cohort differences between different age groups, such as 65–69 years, 70–74 years, 75–84 years, 85–94 years, and 95+ years.*
2. *Identify at least three different trends in the population noted in the 2010 census within the aging population as compared with older adults at different points in history.*
3. *Compare and contrast similarities and differences in education, health, housing, and marital status across different age cohorts.*
4. *Analyze and identify some differences in expectations in long-term care and community care practices for groups of older adults across different age cohorts that you will be confronted with as a health care or social services provider.*
5. *Describe your vision for an ideal living environment when you reach age 65, 75, 85, and 95.*

REFERENCES

Administration on Aging, U.S. Department of Health and Human Services. (2001). Retrieved May 26, 2012 from http://www.aoa.gov/aoaroot/aging_statistics/Profile/2011/docs/2011profile.pdf

Federal Interagency Forum on Aging-Related Statistics. (2010). Retrieved December 11, 2011 from http://www.fedstats.gov/key_stats/index.php?markup=XHTML&pageType=program&id=health

Hogan, H., Perez, D., & Bell, W. R. (2008). Who (really) are the first Baby Boomers? In *Joint Statistical Meetings Proceedings, social statistics section* (pp. 1009–1016). Alexandria, VA: American Statistical Association.

Jurkowski, E. T. (2008). *Policy and program planning for older adults: Visions and realities*. New York, NY: Springer Publishing.

Kapp, M. (2012, May 14). How to fix nursing homes. *The Atlantic*. Retrieved from www.theatlantic.com/health/archive/2012/05/how-to-fix-nursing-homes/257153

National Center for Health Statistics for Older Adults, The Centers for Disease Control and Prevention. (2010). Retrieved from: http://www.cdc.gov/nchs/nchs_for_you/older_americans.htm

Schoeneman, K., & Bowman, C. (2006). *Development of the Artifacts of Culture Change Tool: Report of Contract HHSM-500-2005-00076P* (Technical report). Baltimore, MD: Centers for Medicaid & Medicare Services. Retrieved from www.artifactsofculturechange.org/Data/Documents/artifacts.pdf

U.S. Census Bureau (2010). *Current Population Survey, Annual Social and Economic Supplement*.

U.S. Census 2010. Retrieval from http:www.census.gov.

Werner, C. A. (2011). *The Aging population. 2010: 2010 Census briefs*. Retrieved May 25, 2012 from: http://www.census.gov/prod/cen2010/briefs/c2010br-09.pdf

Werner, C. (2011, November). The older population: 2010. *2010 Census Briefs*. Retrieved from www.census.gov/prod/cen2010/briefs/c2010br-09.pdf

Wolfensberger, W. (1972). *The principle of normalization in human services*. Toronto, ON, Canada: National Institute on Mental Retardation.

Wolfensberger, W. (1980). The definition of normalization: Update, problems, disagreements and misunderstandings. In R. J. Flynn & K. E. Nitsch (Eds.), *Normalization, social integration and human services* (pp. 71–115). Baltimore, MD: University Park Press.

2

Introduction to Long-Term Care Settings and Culture Change

To the novice working in the field of long-term care, the myriad options available for care settings may appear to be both daunting and difficult to understand. This chapter is designed to provide an overview of the various types of long-term care settings and to help readers understand how these settings are similar or differ. Readers who are seasoned veterans of the long-term care setting arena may utilize this chapter as a primer for the new employees, certified nursing assistants, nurses, or social service workers who join their facility. Ideally, the chapter helps provide a context not only for the setting in which they are newly employed, but also for the range of settings within the long-term care continuum.

THE EVOLUTION OF LONG-TERM CARE SETTINGS

Long-term care and the various options available for residential and long-term care settings for older adults have evolved over time and have arrived into the settings as we know them today in the 21st century. Ironically, only about 5% of the U.S. population today reside in nursing care settings. Prior to the 18th century, however, no specific institutions for long-term care existed, and those that did exist incorporated care for people with disabilities, people who were frail and/or elderly, and individuals considered either deviant or insane by their communities. These settings, which were developed on the basis of the concept of almshouses, originated from England via the Elizabethan Poor Laws of 1601. The Elizabethan Poor Laws granted the state responsibility for ensuring the care of the needy, hungry, isolated, and infirm. The laws sanctioned the state to assume responsibility for individuals and their care when family, social supports, and religious communities were not available to assist a person in need (de Sweinitz, 1943).

According to the Elizabethan Poor Laws, elderly individuals in need of shelter or who were incapacitated, impoverished, or isolated from their families, could be placed in almshouses as an alternative to living on the street without resources. However, at times elderly people in such situations were treated rather inhumanely. They were often forced into care situations along with people diagnosed with mental illness, substance abuse issues, and/or intellectual deficits, and those who were homeless. Thus, the culture of treatment and care for elderly individuals was less than ideal, and it certainly did not take into consideration concepts such as self-determinism, empowerment, or the least restrictive environment.

In some instances, the Catholic Church developed homes for the infirm and aged, and took in and cared for older adults as a part of its mission to provide service to the community. Currently there are many nursing homes and long-term care settings that provide skilled nursing care to people who are physically disabled and in need of nursing care (these will be more clearly defined and differentiated later in this chapter). Although the trend is for these same facilities to be operated under a secular board of directors, their roots emerged from the Elizabethan Poor Laws.

Early in the 19th century, a rise in the number of special homes to care for elderly people emerged in the United States. These homes emerged through women's organizations and church groups and were intended to address the needs of elderly people in the community. Although these homes likely were developed out of a concern that worthy people within their own ethnic or religious background might be forced into care situations alongside people who were considered indigent and therefore despised, they at least offered an alternative to the care available at the time. "As the founder of Boston's Home for Aged Women (1850), explained—[these homes were] a haven for those who were 'bone of our bone, and flesh of our flesh'" (Public Broadcasting Service, 2012). Advocates for these homes contrasted the benevolent care they provided with the horrors experienced by people who were relegated to almshouses. "We were grateful," wrote the organizers of Philadelphia's Indigent Widows' and Single Women's Society, one of the nation's earliest old age homes, in 1823, "that through the indulgence of

Divine Providence, our efforts have, in some degree, been successful, and have preserved many who once lived respectfully from becoming residents of the Alms House" (*The History of Nursing Homes*, 2012).

It is not surprising that, because of stringent regulations, high fees for care and supervision, and the "certificates of good character" that were required for admission, few aging people in the communities were admitted into these homes. Those who were admitted tended to be widowed and single women who had spent their lifetimes in service for their community. The state of Massachusetts reported that 2,598 people were housed in these facilities in 1910.

Given that the majority of older adults would not qualify for shelter in these facilities, another type of almshouse emerged in the early 1900s. These publicly owned facilities, known as *poor farms*, were for the most part unregulated and considered to be a place of last resort for people who had no other caregiver options. The elderly individuals and people with disabilities who lived in these situations faced horrifying living conditions. These horrifying living conditions included isolation, limited nursing or personal care, and limited nutrition and hydration. These poor farms did not benefit from any federal assistance programs to help pay for or subsidize care. It appears that the states, rather than trying to provide assistance to older adults in a dignified manner, encouraged the dilapidated conditions and facilities, along with inadequate care, as a strategy to promote a stigma against their use (Allen, 2008; Lehning & Austin, 2010).

In the meantime, by 1920, hospitals began to change their image to "houses of hope." Previously, they had been perceived as places where people died or where people sought their last refuge or as sanctuaries for the poor (Lehning & Austin, 2010).

The New Deal, formulated in the early 1930s, promoted the idea that older adults should receive benefits on the basis of need rather than as a universal benefit. This concept was short lived, and the stigma that had existed against people of advancing age came back to the forefront of society with the passage of the Social Security Act of 1935. One of the provisions of this piece of legislation was that it banned people in public facilities from receiving any form of "Old Age Assistance." The Act, signed into legislation by then-President Franklin Delano Roosevelt on August 14, 1935, provided states with financial resources in the form of matching grants called *Old Age Assistance* (OAA) to retired workers. As a strategy to discourage residence in almshouses, people who did live in these settings were not allowed to receive OAA benefits. This regulation led to the development of care facilities known as *private old-age homes*. The development of these homes allowed people to continue to receive care and still collect OAA payments.

The Hospital Survey and Reconstruction Act of 1946 (also known as the Hill–Burton Act) paved the way for funding the construction of state-of-the-art community hospitals. Despite the passage of this legislation, the events of the Great Depression and World War II created a tremendous backlog of facilities in need of upgrade, including many community hospitals. Thus, long-term care facilities for the elderly and infirm became less of a priority.

The regulations within the Social Security Act limited OAA payments to private old age homes as opposed to almshouses, and thus paved the way for the disappearance of the almshouses. Some argue that this was a strategy to eliminate almshouses altogether. During this same era, public hospital associations continued to lobby Congress, resulting in amendments to the Social Security program and new legislation in support of older adults. The Medical Facilities Survey and Construction Act of 1954 provided for the development of nursing facilities and thus attempted to improve the care older adults received by facilitating the construction of such facilities in conjunction with a hospital. This legislation can be perceived as a landmark in the history of long-term care for two reasons. First, because long-term care facilities were directed to be built alongside hospitals, the facilities began to be framed with a medical model perspective (a topic more fully defined in Chapter 3), and a pathway was created whereby nursing homes would be built and molded more like hospitals. Second, this legislation moved nursing home care from the welfare state/human service system into the health care realm. Before this time, nursing care for older adults had followed the path led by the Elizabethan Poor Laws and almshouses, which were part of the welfare state rather than the health care system.

During this same time frame, practices were being called into question about the care and treatment of people with disabilities and people with defined psychopathologies or mental illnesses. The advent of psychotropic medications began to lay the groundwork for people who had previously been institutionalized to move into community care settings. In addition, advances in the fields of mental impairment led advocacy groups to push for support toward community-based options for their loved ones who had been diagnosed with some form of intellectual or cognitive deficiency. Thus, during the Kennedy Administration, two task forces were developed to explore solutions and identify strategies for alternate care models that would replace the current substandard institutions, almshouses, and care options. The President's Commission on Mental Retardation and the President's Commission on Mental Illness were convened in 1963 to explore options and provide recommendations to the President regarding programming, policy, and practice for these populations. These included recommendations for community-based care, residential living, and vocational training. Programs such as community-independent living arrangements, group home models, and apartment support programs all originated from the recommendations made during these commissions (President's Commission on Mental Retardation, 1963; President's Commission on Mental Illness, 1963).

Amendments to the Social Security program, which took place in 1965 with the passage of programs such as Medicare and Medicaid, added to continued growth among nursing homes and the nursing home industry. President Lyndon B. Johnson's historic speech helps one understand the mindset that led to the reforms signed into legislation in 1965:

> Thirty years ago, the American people made a basic decision that the later years of life should not be years of despondency and drift. The result was enactment of our Social Security program ... Compassion and reason dictate that this logical extension of our proven Social Security system will supply the prudent, feasible, and dignified way to free the aged from the fear of financial hardship in the event of illness (The history of nursing homes, 2012).

Legislative changes continued to play a role in the development of nursing homes. For example, in 1968 Congress passed legislation to provide improvements in nursing homes and raise the standards of care within them. This legislation, known as the Moss Amendments, help set the stage for increased standards of care in and promoted regulatory control in long-term care facilities (Allen, 2008).

In April 1969, in response to the skyrocketing costs among beneficiaries, Medicare stopped providing coverage for long-term care. The Department of Health and Human Service issued an *intermediary letter 371* (a term used to convey changes to the federal rules or regulations) that negated much of the original coverage for nursing homes that the Medicare program had initially allowed. The end result was that older adults and their families were left with exorbitant bills that were beyond the scope of what average families could afford.

In response to this dramatic change in the shift in Medicare coverage, intermediate-care facilities were born. With most nursing homes across the country unable to comply with the standards set by the government, the Miller Amendment offered states an alternative to the costly changes (Allen, 2008). It established a new standard: intermediate-care facilities. This new classification meant the facility qualified for federal reimbursement but did not require the same amount of skilled nursing or resources, thus costing the government less and lowering standards of care.

Beginning in 1971, therefore, policymakers began to enact numerous government regulations in order to control the quality of long-term care. In 1971, the Office of Nursing Home Affairs provided a structure to oversee numerous agencies responsible for nursing home standards. In 1972, reforms of Social Security legislation established a single set of requirements for facilities supported by Medicare and for skilled-nursing homes that received Medicaid. Although this limited the ability of most individuals to enter skilled-nursing facilities, it increased the demand for intermediate-care facilities. Other amendments to the Older American Act in 1973 and 1987 provided and strengthened statewide nursing home ombudsman programs. Nursing homes residents and their families now had a secure way of voicing any institutional complaints.

Between 1960 and 1976, the number of nursing homes grew by 140%, the number of nursing home beds increased by 302%, and the industry's revenues rose by 2000%. To a great extent, this growth was stimulated by private industry. By 1979, despite the ability of government homes to provide care, 79% of all institutionalized elderly persons resided in commercially run homes (Administration on Aging, 2012).

According to investigations of the industry in the 1970s, many of these institutions provided substandard care. Lacking the required medical care, food, and attendants, they were labeled "warehouses" for the old and "junkyards" for the dying by numerous critics. In 1972, Medicaid began covering the costs of long-term care for people with little income and few resources. Other landmark pieces of legislation included the Boren Amendment, passed in 1981, a federal law that required states to ensure "reasonable and adequate" provider reimbursement rates. This law was enforceable by the federal courts.

The Institute of Medicine published a report in 1985 that examined the impact of nursing home regulation. This report became the basis for the legislation contained in the Omnibus Reconciliation Act, which in 1987 provided for an overhaul of regulations for nursing homes. Included within this legislation was the Nursing Home Reform Act, part of which established quality standards for nursing homes and illuminated the need for quality of life and the preservation of residents' rights. The Nursing Home Reform Act spurred a group of long-term care advocates to band together to transform the nursing home and long-term care environments and create a change of the current culture known to nursing home residents. From their actions, the concept of "culture change" emerged (Doty, Koren, & Sturla, 2008).

In the 1990s, the concept of subacute care, a strategy to provide care to people who had been released from hospitals but still needed more care than was available in intermediate care nursing facilities, emerged. Despite rapid growth in Medicare nursing home expenditure, the Balanced Budget Act cut the amount of money Medicare paid to nursing homes. This had a huge impact on the funding stream available to nursing home networks, bankrupting several nursing home chains and almost bankrupting many others. In addition to this, the Boren Amendment was repealed. Both of these activities occurred in 1997 and led to a shift in vision and practice for nursing home care through the lens of an institutionalized care model.

These policies, however, did not uniformly raise the standards of all nursing homes; neither did they eliminate the fear expressed by many older adults who faced a nursing-home admission with dread. Yet, as the percentage of the oldest-old population (i.e., over age 85) has continued to grow, nursing home care has become an increasing reality for many. By 2000, nursing homes had become a $100 billion industry, paid largely by Medicaid, Medicare, and out-of-pocket expenses, and although only 2% of all elderly individuals between age 65 and 74 reside in such institutions, the proportion of those over 85 increased to 25% (National Clearinghouse on Long Term Care Information, 2012).

The medical model approach found in nursing home settings was challenged in the late 1980s by Dr. Bill Thomas, who wanted to shift from a model of institutionalized care to one of care with human connections and caring. He advocated the *Eden Alternative*, a philosophy of culture change built around a set of 10 principles that focus on eliminating the three plagues of loneliness, helplessness, and boredom for elders. Created in 1994 by Bill Thomas and Jude Thomas, the Eden Alternative has grown to become the most practiced approach to culture change in the world.

One part of the Eden Alternative is the *Green House Model*, in which long-term care residences shifted from large-scale care facilities to smaller household communities of older adults who need either skilled nursing care or assisted living care. These communities generally were composed of people in groups of 10 or fewer (6–10 people) who required care, with a focus on quality of life rather than on the illness and limitations of the residents.

The Eden Alternative approach to quality of life and person-centered care inspired a group of long-term care advocates who wanted to infuse many of the same principles of care and a person-centered approach to long-term care settings to join forces. They called themselves *pioneers in long-term care*. Through a series of collaboration discussions between Dr. Thomas and other pioneers who were trying to cultivate a different approach to providing long-term care to frail elders, the culture change movement evolved (Misiorski, 2004; Pioneer Network, 1997). This national movement set the stage for the transformation of services and facilities available to older adults requiring nursing care through institutional settings. This culture change approach is based on a core set of values such as dignity, choice, respect, and self-determination.

The nursing home leaders who initiated the culture change movement are known today as the *Pioneers* (Pioneer Network, 1997), but the group is still in early stages of development (Rahman & Schnelle, 2008). The grassroots culture change movement (which included Dr. Bill Thomas) established a mission and vision for what is known today as the *Pioneer Network culture change movement*. This group's vision included the transformation of long-term care residential settings into homelike settings in which individual dignity and choice were valued and that had a person-centered focus, as opposed to an institutional setting (Pioneer Network, n.d.).

In 2000, the Centers for Medicaid & Medicare Services, under the leadership of Karen Schoerneman and Carmen Bowman, developed an instrument designed to help managers of long-term care residences assess their facilities within six domains in an effort to help create a baseline for their transformative efforts and lay the groundwork for planned transformation. The six domains, (a) care practices, (b) environmental practices, (c) leadership, (d) family, (e) community, and (f) outcomes, are all elements of the organizational practice and culture within care settings. Although sweeping changes have taken place over the past decade, much work is still required on transformational efforts to create systemic change and address the person-centered needs that people present.

This chapter thus far has attempted to provide a history of the development of nursing homes and long-term care for people who are growing older. It has attempted also to showcase some of the developments within these facilities. Ideally, with the type of legislation enacted, it is clear where the concept of "sterility" within the long-term care environment originated. In addition, it is hoped that the emergence of different strategies for care has been differentiated. The concepts of intermediate-care, subacute care, and rehabilitative care may be new to some readers, so the next section addresses each of these options for care and outlines how they are similar to or different from each other.

LONG-TERM CARE SETTINGS

A range of long-term care settings are available to people advancing in age and people with disabilities. These options include independent living, assisted living, intermediate-care facilities, skilled nursing care facilities, rehabilitation facilities, naturally occurring retirement communities, continuing care communities, adult foster care facilities, board-and-care facilities, and subacute care facilities. For the novice, this list may seem daunting and leave one wondering how one differentiates each option. The following sections outline each of these options and identify some of the salient features of each option. To help conceptualize the differences, we consider three distinctions: (a) independent living, (b) supportive/shelter care, and (c) nursing home care.

Independent Living Options

Independent Living

Independent living is a general name for any housing arrangement designed exclusively for seniors. Other terms include *retirement communities, retirement homes, senior housing,* and *senior apartments*. These may be apartment complexes, condominiums, or even free-standing homes. In general, the housing is friendlier to older adults, tends to be compact, and includes help with outside maintenance. Sometimes recreational centers or clubhouses are available on site. This independent living option is available to people 55 years and older who have the capacity to care for themselves. In general, within senior-oriented communities a service coordinator will check in routinely to ensure that no needs are unmet and to help facilitate independence. Some retirement communities offer various additional supportive services for a fee.

Assisted Living

In general, assisted living is a housing option for persons who need help with some activities of daily living, including minor help with medications. Costs tend to vary according to the level of daily help required, although staff are generally available 24 hours a day. Some assisted living facilities provide apartment-style living with scaled-down kitchens, and others provide only rooms. Most facilities have a group dining area and common areas for social and recreational activities.

Assisted living facilities are an apartment-style habitat designed to focus on providing assistance with daily living activities. They provide a higher level of service, including meal preparation, housekeeping, medication assistance, and laundry, and staff also do regular check-ins on the residents. They have been designed to bridge the gap between independent living and nursing home facilities. Often the facilities are equipped with emergency signaling devices. All residents use shared spaces, which usually include living rooms, dining rooms, and/or laundry rooms. Minimal services, ranging from central dining programs to organized recreational activities, health care, transportation, housekeeping, nonpersonal laundry, and security are included in most plans for assisted living. In general, a licensed care staff and physician are not on duty routinely within these facilities.

There are more than 26 designations that states use to refer to what is commonly known as *assisted living*. There is no single uniform definition of assisted living, and there are no federal regulations that govern assisted living facilities. In many states, most assisted living is private pay, although some states, such as Illinois, have developed a Medicaid waiver program to assist with the costs of living in these facilities for people living below the poverty line.

The Village Concept

The village solution to aging in place is a relatively new concept, enabling active seniors to remain in their own homes without having to rely on family and friends. Members of a "village" can access specialized programs and services, such as transportation to the grocery store, home health care, or help with household chores, as well as a network of social activities with other village members. As of 2009, there were 50 village organizations across the United States. Each offers different services depending on the local needs of the individual communities. The cost of membership varies according to geographic area and the level of services required, but is often in excess of $500 a year.

Naturally Occurring Retirement Communities

Like the village concept, naturally occurring retirement communities enable seniors to stay in their own homes and access local services, volunteer programs, and social activities, but they tend to exist in lower income areas. A naturally occurring retirement community may be as small as a single urban high rise or spread out over a larger suburban area.

Continuing-Care Retirement Facilities

Continuing-care retirement communities are facilities that include independent living, assisted living, and nursing home care in one location, so seniors can stay in the same general area as their housing needs change over time. This type of care normally involves the cost of buying a unit in the community as well as monthly fees that increase as higher levels of care are required. This option is attractive to people who would like to stay in the same general facility regardless of care needs. It also allows spouses to be close to one another even if one requires a higher level of care. Within these communities a number of services are available, including in-home services. In-home services allow an individual to continue to live in his or her residence while receiving help with activities such as meal preparation, shopping, and/or nursing care. Depending on the circumstances, the services provided range from minimal (e.g., housekeeping, shopping, conversation) to extensive help with activities of daily living (bathing, dressing, taking medication, etc.). Continuing-care retirement communities, also called *multilevel care facilities*, provide a nice balance among a skilled-nursing home, assisted living facility, and an independent living facility or retirement community. It ensures that the recipient maintains independent living as long as possible, while providing for nursing assistance if or when it is needed.

These facilities offer many services, including personal conveniences (hairdresser/barber, banks, library), organized social and recreational activities, educational programs, exercise classes, craft and woodworking activities, gardening space, transportation, and health care. Because these activities can be costly, the entrance fee and monthly charges are often quite large. In addition, entrance restrictions normally specify a minimum age, as well as a minimum level of health and finances. Entrance lists for such facilities are often months or years long.

Supportive/Shelter Care Options

Congregate Care

Congregate care living is very similar to independent living complexes. It has the aspects of a community environment, with one or more meals per day prepared and served in a community dining hall. Private quarters are allowed, and the services and amenities provided can include transportation, pools, a convenience store, bank, barber/beauty shop, resident laundry, housekeeping, and security.

Group Homes

Group homes provide an independent living environment with only minimal services. These services are much like those offered in an independent living facility. Group homes differ, however, in that the individual usually co-owns or rents the home with a group of individuals who share the common areas of the living environment.

Residential Care Facilities

Residential care facilities, also called *board-and-care homes, personal care homes, sheltered housing,* or *domiciliary care homes,* offer housing for individuals who need assistance with personal care or medical needs. This means that the facility is normally state licensed and meets minimum staffing requirements. The facility is staffed 24 hours a day. To be eligible for residential care facilities, an individual usually must be fairly mentally alert; able to dress, feed, and take him- or herself to the toilet; able to eat meals in a central dining room; and need no more than moderate assistance with personal care or behavior supervision. Potential residents should check with the specific facility for any policies concerning walkers or wheelchairs.

These facilities usually feature studio or one-bedroom apartments that lack kitchens but have private bathrooms and storage units. Some facilities offer only shared rooms, which can be a difficult adjustment for many. Additional services include meals, social activities, laundry, and housekeeping services.

Adult Foster Care

Adult foster care options generally match people who are not capable of living independently or safely on their own with a foster family. The family provides room and board round the clock for 24 hours per day along with help with personal care activities such as bathing, feeding, and medication management. Foster families generally take one person or a small group of adults into their residence. This option is generally licensed by the state, and the name (i.e., *adult foster care*) may vary from location, region or state.

Board-and-Care Homes

Two main types of board-and-care homes exist: (a) a residential care facility and (b) a group home. The distinction between the two lies within the number of residents for which the home is licensed. Residential facilities, for example, have 20 or fewer residents, whereas group homes will have six or fewer residents. The rooms may be shared or private, and nursing and medical services are generally not provided. Both types of facilities provide meals, personal care, and staff available around the clock. This option is generally licensed by the state, and the name (i.e., *board and care*) may not be consistent across state lines.

Nursing Home Care Options

A nursing home is normally the highest level of care for older adults outside of a hospital. Although they do provide assistance in activities of daily living, they differ from other senior housing in that they also provide a high level of medical care. A licensed physician supervises each resident's care, and a nurse or other medical professional is almost always on the premises. Skilled nursing care and medical professionals, such as occupational or physical therapists, are also available.

Nursing home care options and the range of services within this network can vary by the type of facility. In general, all facilities will provide housing and housekeeping duties. At the nursing home care level, assistance usually is provided with managing medication, personal care and supervision, and 24-hour nursing care under the supervision of a physician. In the case of people with Alzheimer's disease, special programs and options may be available. In addition, the facility is often licensed and the constellation of services offered is regulated by the state in which it is located. For example, some states do not allow some types of facilities to include residents who are wheelchair bound or who cannot exit the facility on their own if there is an emergency. Nursing homes also provides meals, assistance with activities of daily living, and recreational activities for residents. Most residents in these homes have physical or mental impairments of such a nature that they can't safely live alone.

The availability of a range of options exist for nursing care. Thus, in this next segment, these options are described. Options for nursing home care include intermediate-care facilities, skilled care, subacute care, rehabilitation, hospice care, and adult day care (Family Care Forum, 2012).

Intermediate Care

Intermediate care when presented as a nursing home care option is designed to meet the needs of people advancing in age or people with disabilities, who need assistance with one or more activities of daily living (ADLs). Despite the fact that there is a need to attend to the individuals' ADLs, residents typically do not have any major or compelling nursing requirements. This type of care is usually requested by a physician and administered by a nurse with a minimum of a "registered nurse" level of training.

Skilled Nursing

Skilled nursing homes or facilities are nursing home facilities or in home care that have been traditionally characterized and associated with nursing home facilities. They provide around the clock medical nursing services for seniors with serious illnesses or disabilities. These facilities are the best option for individuals who need 24-hour medical supervision, skilled nursing care, and/or rehabilitation.

This level of care includes help with more complex nursing tasks, such as monitoring medications, giving injections, caring for wounds, and providing nourishment by tube feedings (enteral feeding). It also includes therapies, such as occupational, speech, respiratory, and physical therapy.

Although this care is most often delivered within a nursing home facility, it is also possible to provide skilled nursing care to someone who is living within their own home. Most insurance plans require at least some level of skilled care need, requiring the services of a licensed professional (e.g., a nurse, doctor, or therapist) before they will cover other home-care services within a skilled nursing facility or one's own home.

Rehabilitation services are provided on a time-limited basis for individuals in need of short-term rehabilitation or a bridge between their hospital stay and a return to home. People who have had hip or knee replacements, for example, may fit into this model of care, because it involves a short-term stay. A request by a physician is generally required for admission to these facilities. The state and federal governments have to license these facilities in order for them to provide care by registered nurses, licensed practical nurses, and certified nursing assistants. These rehabilitation services generally are designed to help restore functional abilities (mental and physical) that have been lost because of an accident or some form of acute illness.

Subacute Care

This option provides care and/or monitoring after one's hospitalization, usually within a less expensive or costly setting than the hospital. The forms of care can include rehabilitation services in a nursing home or a stay, usually short-term, in a specialized unit within a hospital.

Acute Care Services

Acute care services address health issues that have recently developed, quickly got worse, or resulted from a recent accident. The primary goal of acute care services is to provide recovery through a short-term stay. The services primarily provided through an acute care scheme include physicians, physician assistants, nurse practitioners, nurses, or other skilled professionals offering short-term medical services.

Custodial Care

Custodial care is yet another option available within nursing home settings. Individuals receiving custodial care need supervision with personal care and other daily living activities but do not require the help of a practical nurse. Individuals with dementia, including Alzheimer's disease, are often given this type of care.

Hospice Care

Hospice care is an infusion of home care and facility care provided to benefit terminally ill patients and support their families through their tough times. This option can be offered within a long-term care facility, and it is covered through Medicare. Hospice care can also be provided directly in the patient home. Medicare will provide funding for this option if a physician indicates that a person probably has 6 months or less to live.

The hospice care program also offers medical and social support/services to people who have been diagnosed with a terminal disease. The approach to hospice care is one that emphasizes "comfort care" through pain control and symptom management. Social support is offered to the individual and his or her family during the time leading up to the person's passing, and grief counseling is often offered to family members for several months postmortem. At the current time, grief counseling and supportive services are not extended to the nursing home staff who provide care to the individual who has passed.

Adult Day Care

Adult day care programs work just like any other day care program. Adult day care programs provide services during the day while the regular caregiver is at work or having a respite. The services can be offered in a nursing facility or a separate facility. The program provides meals, structured activities, and care services to seniors in a community or within a nursing facility during the day, for a specific time period during the day. In general, the people who attend adult day care services are in need of social interactions and have some level of cognitive and functional impairments.

Respite Care

Respite care is offered only on a temporary basis. It allows the primary caregiver or family member relief for a few days, or even just a few hours. Respite care can be delivered through a nursing facility or assisted living facility. Respite care can be delivered also through several different venues and covered through different funding mechanisms. A home health worker can come into one's home for short-term assistance, or a person may be admitted for short-term respite care to a long-term care facility. Funding for respite care is available through local home health providers, funded through the Older Americans Act, or through Medicare for in facility respite stays (Family Care America, 2012).

Regardless of the setting for care, there is no guarantee that the services will be delivered with a person-centered approach (i.e., that the person's needs are placed before the task at hand). As discussed earlier in this chapter, the notion that long-term care facilities were aligned with hospitals paved the way for long-term care settings to take on the features of a hospital environment—that is, one of sterility that embraces a medicalized approach to the provision of care. With this view in mind, it becomes easier to understand why long-term care settings have been set up to function like a medical facility rather than a home. Some facilities within the disability network have had a longer tradition of considering the person first and may not be as entrenched in the medical approach to care. However, there still may be room for changes and advances so that the home/facility can more strongly reflect a culture of personal affirmation rather than a culture of sterility.

This chapter reviewed some of the history behind long-term care settings and explored some of the different options for community and institutional living for people advancing in age or living with a disability. The next chapter explores different philosophical paradigms to care for people advancing in age or people with disabilities so that readers can more clearly understand the concepts related to personhood and culture change.

DISCUSSION/REFLECTION QUESTIONS

1. *Compare and contrast the early approaches to care for people who are advancing in age and people with disabilities to the approaches that have evolved over the past 25 years.*
2. *Discuss the shift between the provision of care via the welfare state and the health care industry. What are the strengths and deficits of each approach in the long term care arena?*
3. *Describe how major pieces of legislation, such as the New Deal, Medicare, and the Omnibus Reconciliation Act, have shaped the culture of long-term care settings.*
4. *Identify which type of care you would prefer for yourself and/or your loved ones and explain why these are your preferences.*

REFERENCES

Administration on Aging. (2012). *Services and providers.* National Clearinghouse on Long Term Care Information. Retrieved from www.longtermcare.gov/LTC/Main_Site/Understanding/Services

Allen, J. E. (2008). *Nursing home administration*. New York, NY: Springer Publishing.
de Sweinitz, K. (1943). *England's road to social security: From the Statute of Laborers in 1349 to the Beveridge Report of 1942*. New York, NY: A. S. Barnes.
Doty, M. M., Koren, M. J., & Sturla, E .L. (2008). *Culture change in nursing homes: How far have we come? Findings from The Commonwealth Fund 2007 National Survey of Nursing Homes*. Retrieved from www.commonwealthfund.org/Publications/Fund-Reports/2008/May/Culture-Change-in-Nursing-Homes--How-Far-Have-We-Come--Findings-From-The-Commonwealth-Fund-2007-Nati.aspx
Family Care America. (2012). *An overview of resources for long term care settings*. Retrieved from www.caregiverslibrary.org/caregivers-resources/grp\care-facilities/the-long-term-care-spectrum-article.aspx
Family Care Forum. (2012). *A glossary of long term care settings*. Retrieved from www.helpguide.org/elder/nursing_homes_skilled_nursing_facilities.htm
The history of nursing homes. (2012). Retrieved from www.4fate.org/history.html
Lehning, A. J., & Austin, M. J. (2010). Long-term care in the United States: Policy themes and promising practices. *Journal of Gerontological Social Work, 53*, 43–63.
Misiorski, S. (2004). *Getting started: A pioneering approach to culture change in long term care organizations*. Rochester, NY: The Pioneer Network.
National Clearinghouse on Long Term Care Information. (2012). Retrieved from www.longtermcare.gov/LTC/Main_Site/Understanding/Services/Facility_Based services.aspx
Pioneer Network. (n.d.). *Vision, mission and values*. Retrieved from www.pioneernetwork.net/AboutUs/Values
Pioneer Network. (1997, March). *Meeting of pioneers in nursing home culture change*. Rochester, NY: Author.
President's Commission on Mental Illness. (1963). *A white paper report on the status of people with mental illness: Findings and recommendations*. Baltimore, MD: U.S. Government Printing Office.
President's Commission on Mental Retardation. (1963). *A white paper report on the status of people with mental retardation: Conclusions and recommendations*. Baltimore, MD: U.S. Government Printing Office.
Public Broadcasting Service. (2012). *The evolution of nursing home care in the United States*. Retrieved from www.pbs.org/newshour/health/nursinghomes/timeline.html
Rahman, A. N., & Schnelle, J. F. (2008). The nursing home culture-change movement: Recent past, present, and future directions for research. *The Gerontologist, 48*, 142–148.

3

Philosophical Paradigms Impacting Long-Term Care Settings

Regardless of what professional or occupational discipline to which one belongs, some specific values are at the heart of what and how one practices. These values are guided by some form of philosophical paradigm. Within human service and health/long-term care settings several philosophical paradigms are at play. Consequently, tension may be found at the forefront of multidisciplinary team meetings or decision-making bodies. Often, the tension is not necessarily about differences in opinion, or differences in the way in which people view the problem from their respective discipline; it may lie in the different practitioners' philosophical differences toward care and treatment. The bases for these differences are often variations between different operating paradigms. These paradigms include the medical model, the rehabilitation/disability paradigm, independent living paradigm, the strengths-based paradigm, the Eden Alternative paradigm, and the culture change paradigm. This chapter explores each of these paradigms, compares and contrasts how they play a role in the provision of service delivery and care within health and human service settings, and lays the groundwork for understanding the values and principles of a culture change paradigm. By the end of the chapter, the way different perspectives shape how services are delivered within the multidisciplinary setting, and how one can work with each different perspective to be able to identify strategies to help opposing perspectives embrace one's own philosophy and perspective, will be clear.

THE MEDICAL MODEL

The medical model paradigm is the oldest and most traditional of all philosophical perspectives. Although some literature suggests that it dates back to the time of Robert Koch and Louis Pasteur, I argue that this approach goes even further back, as far as Hippocrates, the father of medicine. Simply put, the medical model focuses on identifying a defect, disease, illness, or dysfunction in the patient. Once one or more deficits have been identified, treatment can be started, and "problem solving," if you will, begins (Mosby, 2009). The basis of the diagnosis is believed to be within the individual, and the deficits may then limit the individual's potential and functioning in the world around him or her. Treatment is based on some way to alter the physical symptoms or their etiology. Neither environment nor human potential is taken into account within the medical model. Physicians have historically used the medical model approach in their professional practice. The field of nursing, however, can differ from the medical model because the patient is perceived as a person relating to the environment holistically, and nursing care is formulated on the basis of a holistic assessment of all dimensions of the person (physical, mental, emotional, and spiritual) that assumes multiple causes for the problems the patient is experiencing. Nursing care thus focuses on all dimensions, not just the physical dimension (Mosby, 2009).

In the field of psychiatry, the medical model views abnormal behavior as the result of physical problems and thus assumes that this behavior should be treated medically. This perspective addresses behavior such as depression, anxiety, or dementias from the view that these conditions are a form of mental illness, and these specific diagnoses are a disease or disease-like condition that can and should be treated through somatic (physical) means by medical personnel, primarily psychiatrists or other types of physicians. The medical model attributes mental illness behaviors to physiological, biochemical, and/or genetic causes and attempts to treat it primarily through physically based (somatic) procedures, in particular, drugs. A mentally ill person is regarded in the medical model in the same manner as anyone with a physical illness. Psychiatric conditions, such as schizophrenia and the affective (mood) disorders, are viewed as similar to physical diseases such as diabetes, epilepsy, and high blood pressure. Physicians (primarily psychiatrists), should be the primary treatment personnel for individuals with mental illness, but other treatment personnel (e.g., nurses, psychologists, and social workers) may also be involved, although in a position of less importance. According to the medical model, the psychiatrist should be the primary decision maker, the overall coordinator of care, and the one who should take primary responsibility for treatment of the patient (Mosby, 2009).

The rise of modern scientific medicine during the 19th century had a great impact on the development of the medical model. Especially important here was the development of the *germ theory* of disease put forth by European medical researchers such as Pasteur and Koch. During the late 19th and early 20th centuries, the physical causes of a variety of diseases were uncovered, a discovery that in turn led to the development of effective forms of treatment. Although much of these medical successes were achieved in the area of physical illness, advances also occurred in the area of "mental" illness as well. For example, in the late 19th century, approximately 20% of all persons hospitalized in mental institutions were actually suffering from a physical disease.

Proper diagnosis (i.e., the categorization of specific signs and symptoms in an effort to identify disease groupings) is a critical component of the medical model. The model assumes that, by using its approach to categorizing signs and symptoms into diagnostic categories, a physician's ability to successfully identify diseases and other physical issues is greatly enhanced. This approach also helps facilitate treatment strategies. Within the medical model accurate diagnosis is important for the following reasons:

1. An accurate diagnosis can help provide the physician with clinically useful information about the course of the illness and/or its prognosis.
2. An accurate diagnosis can point to (or at least suggest) a specific underlying cause or causes for the disorder.
3. An accurate diagnosis can help direct the physician to specific treatment or treatments for the condition.

A major criticism of the medical model by other medical professionals —medical sociologists, for example—is that in some arenas, such as psychiatry, a diagnosis is often based not on objective facts but on a subjective judgment by a psychiatrist and cultural/social biases about what is or is not considered "normal." These two differing points of view constitute one of the main dividing lines between supporters of the medical model and some of the other philosophical perspectives that are discussed in this chapter.

Lastly, subscribing to the medical model can lead to a number of outcomes for the individual patient (or resident) and the broader social milieu, which can be perceived as either positive or negative depending on which side of the aisle one is on and which philosophical perspective one holds. Some of the following are realities within the medical model:

1. The physician assumes an authoritarian position in relation to the patient. Because of the specific expertise of the physician, according to the medical model, this position is necessary and to be expected. The patient is generally seen as passive and dependent on the physician for advice and guidance. If one extends this perspective into the realm of psychiatry, the medical model generally supports the use of involuntary treatment when necessary.
2. The physician views him- or herself as the dominant health care professional. The physician's expertise in matters of disease, diagnosis, and treatment demand that he or she be viewed as the chief decision maker in medical matters (rather than nurses, psychologists, social workers, or others). This approach does not support a team-oriented, multidisciplinary approach to treatment, and it divorces the patient or resident from having voice in the treatment process.
3. A person with some presenting symptoms of illness or disease should not be held responsible for his or her condition and should not be blamed or stigmatized for his or her illness, whether it is depression, high blood pressure, multiple sclerosis, or dementia. This approach, too, divorces patients from responsibility for their own health behavior and preventive health opportunities.
4. It is the disease condition of the patient that is of major importance. Social, psychological, and other external factors that may influence patient behavior may be ignored or de-emphasized. From a medical model point of view, the problem of mental illness (be it schizophrenia, depression, attention-deficit/hyperactivity disorder, or substance abuse) is an individual problem to be treated individually, and not a social problem treated from a social point of view (due to external factors; Jurkowski, 1997).

In summary, the medical model bases the prognosis of individuals and outcome on the basis of the limitations that are imposed because of a person's diagnosis or disease. This perspective may severely limit people who are advancing in age or people with disabilities and mobility limitations because it suggests that they may not function at their optimal level and that treatment of the disorder is the main key. It negates the roles that environment and human potential may play for one's adaptation. In contrast, the other paradigms do take into consideration the human spirit and resilience.

THE REHABILITATION/DISABILITY PARADIGM

The World Health Organization's (2012) *International Classification of Functioning, Disability and Health* takes into account the social aspects of disability and does not see disability only as a medical or biological dysfunction. This approach helps us understand the importance of the rehabilitation/disability paradigm. After the return to the United States of soldiers from World War I, and their return to Canada after World War II, disabled returning veterans were confined to long-term care facilities to protect them from the hardships and cruelties of the outside world (Jurkowski, 1997). It was not long before these veterans, with broken and wounded bodies but active minds, were restless and eager to return to the world around them. Despite their motivation, the diagnoses affiliated with their disability and the approach to treatment bestowed on them by the medical model left them labeled and stigmatized. Their fight for resources to help them return to the community, with retraining and support, led to the development of the rehabilitation/disability paradigm. This paradigm moves beyond the medical model and argues that, with rehabilitation, a person will be able to restore his or her functioning and return to some meaningful activity within the community. The rehabilitation process is time limited, however, and the resources available to the rehabilitation process are finite. Consequently, this paradigm does offer some limitations because it may take some people longer to adapt or move through the grieving process before they can be actively ready for rehabilitation in the event of some loss of function, loss of limbs, paralysis, and so on. Rehabilitation centers or programs in long-term care settings use this approach and will temporally limit treatment and or rehabilitation (Institute of Medicine, 1997). Toward the conclusion of the time frame allotted, the treatment team will assess the candidate's condition and decide whether the outcomes warrant continuation of rehabilitation orientation interventions. Medicare currently limits a bed stay in a rehabilitation unit for up to 6 weeks post subacute incident (Medicare and You, 2012). Some of the problems inherent in this paradigm include the assumptions that disability is perceived as a deficiency or abnormality, that the disability resides in the individual, that the remedy for disability-related problems is the "cure" or "normalization" of the individual, and that the agent of remedy is the professional (physical therapist, occupational therapist, etc.; Pope & Tarlov, 1991).

In summary, although the rehabilitation paradigm does suggest the need for therapy and resources to provide restoration of functioning, the responsibility for the outcome still rests on the individual to make the changes, and it relies on the professional to provide accurate assessments of what therapeutic milieu should be supported. The process still takes into consideration an expert–consumer model as opposed to a partnership between the rehabilitation specialist and the consumer.

THE INDEPENDENT-LIVING PARADIGM

The independent-living paradigm, conceptualized by DeJong (1979), is more than a social movement; it is also an analytic paradigm that has reshaped the thinking of rehabilitation professionals and researchers. This paradigm moves the locus of barrier away from the person with the impairment or disability and transfers it to the environment. It suggests that an individual may not be capable of the rehabilitation or treatment necessary to restore him or her to an able-bodied state but, with the right combination of supports and assistance, can function as an able-bodied individual.

People with disabilities have increasingly championed the "de-medicalization" of disability, arguing that disability is in large measure the result of a social environment that fails to address the needs of individuals with disabilities and claiming that the medical model of disability fosters dependence rather than personal autonomy. "Members of (the independent-living and disability-rights movements) correctly argue that disability is the result of a dynamic process involving complex interactions among biological, behavioral, psychological, social, and environmental factors" (Pope & Tarlov, 1991, p. 82). An example may help readers more readily draw the distinctions between this paradigm and others, such as the medical model and rehabilitation/disability paradigm.

In this example, we will visit Elizabeth, a 35-year-old mother of three children, all under age 8. Elizabeth contracted polyneuritis through a virus and completely lost the use of all limbs after the virus attacked her central nervous system. Her physician and neurologist argued for her to move into a long-term care nursing home because she was not able to perform any of her basic care needs, such as going to the bathroom, bathing, feeding herself, dressing herself, and transferring herself from her bed to her wheelchair. She was determined to return home to her family and parent her children along with her husband. Thus, she engaged in rehabilitation, but some of the residual side effects of the virus left her unable to completely care for herself. Through the vision of her family and therapist, a number of supports were put into Elizabeth's home to ensure that she would be able to live within a least restrictive environment. These supports included family and social networks, environmental changes to accommodate for Elizabeth's mobility limitations, and strategies to support her activities of daily living. Her children turned their support into games, such as feeding strategies.

Considering this scenario, note that buying into the physician's and neurologist's prognosis would have imposed the medical model paradigm on this family's situation. If one had relied solely on the progress made in therapy as a benchmark for when Elizabeth could return to her family, she may have remained in a rehabilitation center for a long time. Alternatively, using the independent living paradigm, Elizabeth's therapist, husband, and children found ways to adapt the environment in order for her to return home and live with her family. This approach allowed Elizabeth and her family to live independently, with dignity and grace.

In summary, the independent living paradigm focuses on building supports and resources within the person's environment to help facilitate his or her ability to function and move about in a setting that offers the least amount of restriction. This approach promotes the integration of an individual within the mainstream environment.

THE STRENGTHS-BASED PARADIGM

The strengths-based paradigm, developed by Saleeby (2008), integrates a social work perspective with a focus on facilitating the use of inherent strengths that people and their families bring to the therapeutic relationship. Through the assessment process, the therapist identifies inherent strengths in a situation and uses these to build resources and strengths as part of the recovery and empowerment process (Saleeby, 2008). This approach attempts to reframe one's perception to find some strengths and to use these strengths to build on a difficult situation. This approach is an empowering alternative to traditional therapies, which typically describe family functioning in terms of psychiatric diagnoses or deficits, or problematic behaviors. This approach also avoids stigmatizing an individual, family, or community through a deficit approach. Using a strengths-based approach is not counterproductive to healing or hope because it leads people toward hope and lets them wrestle with their strengths to build resiliency.

An additional dynamic of this approach is that it is at odds with the "victim identity," which is often epitomized in popular culture by the appearance of individuals on television or talk radio sharing intimate details of their problems—which is inherently self-defeating. The strengths-based approach inventories (often for the first time in the person's experience) the positive building blocks that already exist in his or her environment that can serve as the foundation for growth and change. It reduces the power and authority barrier between the person and therapist by promoting the person to the level of expert in regard to what has worked, what does not work, and what might work in that person's specific situation. This paradigm also works toward diminishing the authoritarian barrier between the client/consumer/resident and the therapist by placing the therapist in the role of partner or guide. Lastly, families are more invested in any process when they feel they are an integral part of it and have a voice in the outcome.

This paradigm also suggests that there is specific language that must be avoided, which is often stigmatizing in the process. Labels that work against a strengths-based approach include words and phrases such as *noncompliant, resistant, unwilling to change, unmotivated, poor insight, dysfunctional, oppositional,* and *defiant*. Within a strengths-based approach, people are never addressed or identified by their diagnosis; instead, they are a person first, followed by a condition.

Rapp, Saleeby, and Sullivan (2005) identified six hallmarks or principles to be used when embracing the strengths-based paradigm in therapeutic practice:

1. Ensure that the therapeutic process is goal oriented.
2. Ensure that the therapeutic process includes a systematic assessment of strengths.
3. Ensure that the environment is rich in resources.
4. Ensure that explicit methods are used for using client and environmental strengths in efforts to attain goals.
5. Build a therapeutic relationship that has an element of hope incorporated into the goal.
6. Ensure that the relationship and goals provide choices that are meaningful for the consumer and that the consumer/client/resident has the authority and opportunity to choose for themselves.

This strengths-based paradigm has shown tremendous promise within the field of social work practice. It is currently a strong modality used and taught among many schools of social work in the United States and Canada. This paradigm builds on the independent living paradigm and helps professionals look at reframing the areas of deficits into areas of strengths in terms of an individual's resources. It also teaches them to embrace environmental barriers and to try to transform the environment or situation rather than the individual.

THE EDEN ALTERNATIVE PARADIGM

Although the Eden Alternative paradigm is not widely disseminated in the literature as a theory per se, its 10 core principles appear to have shaped the culture of long-term care facilities to a great degree. Consequently, I feel it is important to address these within the context of this chapter, because these principles have had a significant impact for the lives of people receiving care in long-term care and institutional settings. The overall mission of the Eden Alternative is "to improve the well-being of elders and their care partners by transforming the communities in which they live and work" (Eden Alternative, 2011). The following are the 10 principles that guide the Eden philosophy:

1. Loneliness, helplessness and boredom account for the majority of suffering among our elders.
2. Life revolves around close and continuing contact with plants, animals and children. It is these relationships that provide the young and old alike with a pathway to life worth living.
3. Loving companionship is the antidote to loneliness. Elders deserve easy access to human and animal companionship.
4. An elder-centered community creates opportunity to give as well as receive care; this is the antidote to helplessness.
5. An elder-centered community imbues daily life with variety and spontaneity by creating an environment in which unexpected and unpredictable interactions and happenings can take place. This is an antidote to boredom.
6. Meaningless activity corrodes the human spirit. The opportunity to do things that we find meaningful is essential to human health.
7. Medical treatment should be the servant of genuine human caring, never its master.
8. An elder-centered community honors its elders by de-emphasizing top-down bureaucratic authority, seeking instead to place the maximum possible decision-making authority into the hands of the elders or into the hands of those closest to them.
9. Creating an elder-centered community is a never-ending process. Human growth must never be separated from human life.
10. Wise leadership is the lifeblood of any struggle against the three plagues. For it there can be no substitute. (Thomas, 1996, p. 5)

These principles and mission appear to be in direct contrast to the medical model paradigm described earlier in this chapter. However, research on facilities that have used these principles has found a number of positive outcomes that have resulted in long-term care facilities embracing this mission and principles. For example, the Texas Long Term Care Institute conducted a 2-year evaluation across six long-term care homes and found outcomes that included a 60% decrease in behavioral incidents, a 48% decrease in staff absenteeism, a 17% decrease in the use of restraints, and an 11% increase in the facility's overall head count, or census. In another study conducted on a facility in Rhode Island, the results revealed that turnover decreased from 46% to 4% and employee injuries were reduced by 63%.

Although the principles and mission of the Eden Alternative are in direct contrast with those espoused by the medical model, research results suggest that a person- and principle-centered approach to care in institutional care facilities may be a positive alternative to consider. The results suggest improved patient outcomes, improved morale on the part of staff, higher residential engagement, and an increased sense of well-being. The Eden Alternative paradigm has been instrumental in laying the groundwork for the culture change paradigm, discussed next.

THE CULTURE CHANGE PARADIGM

The culture change paradigm appears to be in direct contrast to the medical model paradigm. Its mission, developed by a network of pioneers who have been working in the long-term care arena "advocates and facilitates deep system change and transformation in the culture of aging" (Misiorski, 2004, p. 2.7). To achieve this mission, the Pioneer Network attempts to find ways to create environments and residential alternatives that are different from the traditional models of long-term and congregate care. Their vision is to create "a **culture** of aging that is life-affirming, satisfying, humane and meaningful" (Misiorski, 2004, p. 2.7). This philosophy argues that

> in-depth change in systems requires change in governmental policy and regulation; change in the individual's and society's attitudes toward aging and elders; change in elders' attitudes towards themselves and their aging; and change in the attitudes and behavior of caregivers toward those for whom they care. (Misiorski, 2004, p. 1.4)

and refers to this philosophical approach as *culture change*.

This mission and vision is based on a number of foundational principles and values. These values appear to be simple, but yet they are powerful in terms of transforming the traditional culture of care to one that is humane, connected, affirming, and life giving. These include the following:

1. Be familiar with each person that you come in contact with and be aware of something special about that person's background and life's accomplishments;
2. Believe in the notion that each person can and does make a difference;
3. Relationships between people are the fundamental building block of a transformed culture;
4. Respond to one's spirit, as well as mind and body;
5. Embrace the belief that risk taking is a normal part of life;
6. Put the person, and his/her needs, before the task;
7. Embrace the concept that all elders are entitled to self-determination wherever they live;
8. Community is the antidote to institutionalization;
9. Do unto others as you would have them do unto you;
10. Promote the growth and development of all;
11. Shape and use the potential of the environment in all its aspects: physical, organizational, psycho/social/spiritual;
12. Practice self-examination, searching for new creativity and opportunities for doing better; and
13. Recognize that culture change and transformation are not destinations but a journey, always a work in progress (Misiorski, 2004).

In addition, a number of "Residents' Rights," identified through the Office of the Ombudsman of the U.S. Administration on Aging, guide the "person-first" philosophy and include the principles that residents have the following rights:

- To be treated with respect and dignity
- To be free from chemical and physical restraints
- To manage their own finances
- To voice grievances without fear of retaliation
- To associate and communicate privately with any person of their choice
- To send and receive personal mail
- To have personal and medical records kept confidential
- To apply for state and federal assistance without discrimination
- To be fully informed prior to admission of their rights, available services, and all charges and
- To be given advance notice of transfer or discharge.

(Administration on Aging, U.S. Department of Health and Human Services, 2012)

In summary, this culture change paradigm places the center of responsibility or locus of control onto the individual, rather than the professional (as in the medical model), and embraces the strengths of the individual resident or consumer, regardless of the person's limitations, medical condition diagnosis, or disease. It encourages partnership rather than an authoritarian approach to treatment and care. This approach will transform long-term care and community care settings from a sterile institutional approach to a community approach built on mutual respect and relationships. The next chapter introduces tools that can be used to facilitate this process of cultural transformation.

This chapter explored a number of different philosophical paradigms that affect the way health care professionals provide treatment to consumers, clients, and residents. The chapter began by addressing the most traditional approach, the medical model paradigm, and progressed through additional models, including the rehabilitation/disability paradigm, the independent living paradigm, the strengths-based paradigm, the Eden Alternative paradigm, and the culture change paradigm. Each of these paradigms plays a role within the health care delivery system. As a change agent, one can choose which of these paradigms to support and toward which one would like to shift. Transformation of a working or living environment will include an understanding of which paradigms are apparent to the situation and a vision and desire to move toward specific values.

DISCUSSION/REFLECTION QUESTIONS

1. *This chapter has discussed several philosophical perspectives to care for consumers/patients residents in human service and institutional settings. Which of these paradigms does your specific discipline embrace and support? How does this perspective support or conflict with the culture change paradigm?*
2. *In a discussion group of two or three peers, identify the mission and vision of at least three facilities that you have either worked at or become familiar with through an internship rotation. Which philosophical paradigm best describes the mission and vision of these organizations? What philosophical or value perspectives would need to be addressed in order to move toward the culture change paradigm?*
3. *On a piece of paper, list the various disciplines that are part of the multidisciplinary team with which you are currently working. (If you are not working on a team, then work in a group of students, with a member who has been part of a team). Identify which stakeholder embraces which*

specific paradigms, as discussed in this chapter. Identify some strategies that can be used within a team setting to familiarize stakeholders with the culture change paradigm, and any other paradigm of your choice from this chapter.

REFERENCES

Administration on Aging, United States Department of Health and Human Services. (2012). *The long-term care ombudsman program*. Baltimore, MD: Government Printing Office.
DeJong, G. (1979). Independent living: From social movement to analytic paradigm. *Archives of Physical Medicine and Rehabilitation*, 60(10), 435–446.
Eden Alternative. (2011). *Eden Alternative: It can be different!* Rochester, NY: The Eden Alternative Inc.
Institute of Medicine. (1997). *Enabling America: Assessing the role of rehabilitation and engineering*. Washington, DC: National Academies Press.
Jurkowski, E. T. (1997). *Leadership and citizen participation, a cross national comparison*. MI: Dissertation Abstracts, Ann Arbor, MI.
Medicare and You. (2012). Retrieved May 26, 2012 from http://www.medicare.gov/coverage/your-medicare-coverage.html
Misiorski, S. (2004). *Getting started: A pioneering approach to culture change in long term care organizations*. Rochester, NY: The Pioneer Network.
Mosby, E. (2009). *Mosby's medical dictionary*. New York, NY: Elsevier Publishing.
Pioneer Network. (n.d.). *Vision, mission and values*. Retrieved from www.pioneernetwork.net/AboutUs/Values
Pioneer Network. (1997). *Meeting of pioneers in nursing home culture change: March 14–16, 1997*. Rochester, NY: The Pioneer Network.
Pope, A., & Tarlov, A. (1991). *Disability in America: Toward a national agenda for prevention*. Washington, DC: National Academies Press.
Rapp, C., Saleeby, D., & Sullivan, W. P. (2005). The future of a strengths based social work. *Advances in Social Work Practice*, 6(1), 79–90.
Saleeby, D. (2008). *The strengths perspective in social work practice* (5th ed.). Boston, MA: Pearson Publishing.
Thomas, W. (1996). *Life worth living*. Acton, MA: VanderWyk & Burnham.
World Health Organization. (2012). *The international classification of functioning, disability and health*. Retrieved from www.who.int/classifications/icf/en

4

Artifacts of Culture Change: An Overview of Purpose and Measurement Practices

The process of measuring outcomes in long-term care settings has been the subject of much debate and study for at least the past few decades. Much of the initial research on older adults was conducted within institutionalized settings. Many stalwart researchers within the field of long-term care have examined issues such as activities of daily living (Katz, 1970), quality of life (Kane, 2003), and quality environments (Lawton, 2001) and the impact these have on residents in long-term care settings. Secondary data have also been collected through Medicare and Medicaid; these are available through the Centers for Medicaid & Medicare (CMS) and statewide aging planning commissions. These studies and strategies have largely examined outcomes of care and provided descriptive data about the state of specific issues within long-term care settings, especially quality of care. The research largely has fallen short in regard to the exploration of how we can advance what we know about the nature of the long-term care environment and how that environment can be transformed to reflect a more "person-centered approach" in long-term care practice.

As a result of the gap, members of the Pioneer Network convened and tried to identify what practices were germane to the process of a culture that reflect a person-centered approach to care delivery in a long-term care setting. The subsequent development of the Artifacts of Culture Change Tool (ACCT) filled this gap. This chapter describes the purpose and development of this tool and provides an overview of some of the six areas it addresses. By the end of the chapter, readers should be aware of the benchmarks to be addressed and ready to embark upon the diffusion of these indicators addressed through the second part of this book.

ARTIFACTS OF CULTURE CHANGE TOOL DEVELOPMENT

The genesis of the ACCT began with its conceptualization in 2001 by Karen Schoeneman and Mary Pratt of the CMS. At the time, the team was co-project officers of the CMS Quality of Life study, "Measures, Indicators, and Improvement of Quality of Life in Nursing Homes" led by Dr. Rosalie A. Kane of the University of Minnesota (Kane et al., 2004). The instrument was originally developed to serve as an additional proxy measure for quality of life, which had no set of "indicators per se." Schoeneman and Pratt completed an initial draft of the tool and conducted their initial field test in a facility in Pennsylvania and in late 2001 they refined the instrument in collaboration with Kane. Bowman continued the work in 2005 through a contract awarded to her private consulting firm from the CMS, which resulted in the current version, modified by Schoeneman. All items represent actual changes observed by, read by, or reported to the developers and highlighted by the individuals who implemented them as important and effective components of a change culture.

Initially four nationally prominent facilities were recruited to help complete the tool and provide feedback regarding the ease of data collection and comprehensibility of the instructions for each item and the instrument in general. However, only three that had implemented many of the culture change artifacts were selected. Schoeneman and Bowman (2006) personally visited and verified the concrete results of these facilities' culture change efforts, helping establish the instrument's content and construct validity.

THE PURPOSE OF THE ACCT

Overall, the ACCT was designed to collect the major concrete changes that professionals in long-term care settings have undertaken in the areas of resident care and workplace practices, resident self-determination and autonomy, and an improved environment. The tool itself was developed by providers and researchers who first identified specific practices that differ from or have been altered in long-term care facilities that are based on the culture change paradigm, as compared to facilities that operate on the basis of the medical model or another paradigm.

Many stakeholder groups (i.e., coalitions of nursing home providers, area agencies on aging, academics, facility administrators, marketing representatives, etc.) would like to compare facilities that have embraced a culture change paradigm with those that have not, and to examine variables (i.e., deficiencies, quality measures, turnover, etc.) to determine the impact that a culture change paradigm can have on outcomes. It is no surprise that such outcome data would have a tremendous impact for stakeholders in various parts of the system, such as providers, nursing home chains, academics, and the CMS, and would probably be used to advocate for systemic changes. However, before this stage is reached, baseline benchmarks are first not only necessary but are critical. To make these comparisons, Schoeneman and Bowman (2006) suggested that

> It is necessary to first measure the culture changes themselves, in order to array culture changing homes on a continuum of actual changes they have accomplished, rather than lumping together as "culture change homes" all homes that indicate they are on the journey of culture change (Schoeneman & Bowman, 2006, page 5).

The ACCT was developed as a response to this need, that is, the need to measure actual changes along the continuum of practices within specific benchmarks. It was to be used as a strategy to collect concrete artifacts of the culture change process that a long-term care facility may or may not possess or use in practice in its day-to-day operations.

PSYCHOMETRIC PROPERTIES

At the time of this writing, the authors of the ACCT have not had the tool tested for psychometric properties or properties of validity and reliability. The constructs and measures, however, demonstrate strong face and content validity, and they capture the essence of measurement items across settings. The tool appears to have good test–retest reliability. The items are purposely not based on resident or staff interviews, thus making the process of data collection easier and promoting interrater reliability. Tools that are based on consumer interviews or interviews with key stakeholders tend to capture what changes people desire and/or the degree of approval/satisfaction that residents, staff, and stakeholders feel toward their long-term care setting. In contrast, the ACCT seeks to directly capture the actual, concrete changes that have been made within settings, after an initial baseline assessment of a setting has been made. As baby boomers mature, and seek out long-term care settings for both themselves and their elders, the items identified within the domains of the ACCT are becoming increasingly interesting to this group. The benchmarks and items identified within the ACCT represent practices that consumers are seeking within long-term care settings. The domains encompassed by the ACCT include care practices, the environment, family and community practices, leadership practices, and workplace practices and outcomes, each of which addresses very specific benchmarks and practices (Schoeneman & Bowman, 2006). Private rooms versus shared and greater levels of autonomy are two of the specific practices included in this instrument because they are of interest to those consumers seeking long-term care settings.

The ACCT was developed not with the intention of replacing any available tools but rather to build on the existing complement of instruments and to add to them an assessment instrument that would document actual policy and facility changes being made by many innovators within the culture change movement. The change process represents an alteration of philosophy and paradigm that will reflect a change in heart, mind, and attitude.

The change process includes vision and leadership on the part of administration, and these two elements are not always visible within the normal day-to-day care expectations that residents and their families experience. The results of vision and leadership are concrete changes facilities make that demonstrate the principles that underpin the heart of the culture change paradigm. Such changes are the markers and artifacts of the change in philosophical perspective that will take place as administrators move their settings from an institutional mindset and begin the journey to create a homelike setting (Schoeneman & Bowman, 2006).

PERSPECTIVES REGARDING THE ACCT

A number of key points and features distinguish the ACCT from other tools, in both its development and implementation, and deserve mention. These specific features include the following:

1. The ACCT was designed to be facilitative rather than punitive and, as such, should not be connected to enforcement or punishment.

It also was not developed for the intention of use by surveyors for data collection purposes. Although the tool provides powerful data on a variety of nursing practices, it was not intended to be used by external facility survey teams to cite deficiencies within facilities.
2. The ACCT was developed through the use of government resources and is in the public domain. People may use the tool freely for its intended purpose, although credit should be given to the source.
3. The ACCT encompasses a concrete set of changes that long-term care facilities make in regard to institutional practice and organizational policies, transforming their culture from an institutional one into one that resembles a homelike setting and that supports the concept of resident empowerment and facilitates the residents' direction and autonomy within their lives.
4. The ACCT is designed to enable staff to gauge and identify their progress and carry out their benchmarking of where they are on the culture change journey.
5. The ACCT is a data collection instrument meant to reflect progress by following a calculation of points and by structuring these points toward total change, partial change, or no change for specific items.
6. The ACCT is a CMS-developed product. As such, it is to remain in its final form but can be given away freely. If the administrators of a facility choose to use the ACCT as part of their organizational practices, it should be used in the form presented, without changes made. A copy of the instrument is available at the conclusion of this chapter.
7. The ACCT was developed on the basis of a review of current research and provider literature, as well as personal discussions with several culture change leaders and their facilities, a series of focus groups conducted within long-term care facilities and input from behavioral scientists and academics working within long-term care initiatives.

FUTURE DIRECTIONS OF THE ACCT

Both the domain and the specific items within each ACCT domain that Schoeneman and Bowman (2006) selected are not intended to be an exhaustive list of all the potential changes a facility might implement on the culture change journey. They identified items for the tool that were empirically based and shared by stakeholders to represent areas that needed significant concrete changes, ones that some facilities have successfully implemented. Schoeneman and Bowman also were mindful that there is a limitless future for new innovations to be developed within long-term care networks.

There undoubtedly are facilities that have attempted to build a culture of human dignity long before the culture change or pioneering movement began; therefore, some relevant items may have been developed that currently do not exist on the ACCT. These resources and ideas can, however, contribute to the development of pertinent tools and strategies. In such cases, facilities may want to think retrospectively about the changes they have made and identify how they have made progress over time.

Embracing the culture change paradigm does not necessarily identify the amount of change that has been undertaken. Benchmarking where a particular facility currently is, and how close it is to a perfect score in some areas versus how distant from a perfect score it is in others can be a helpful way for administrators to identify a blueprint for change. When the ACCT was initially conceptualized, its architects envisioned that it would be computerized and made available on a website for any facility to complete easily with programmed computations. At the current time, this resource can be found through the Pioneering Coalition website, with results from participating facilities that have helped with compiling data on outcome scores (see www.pioneernetwork.net/Data/Documents/Tools.pdf). This database and website can be helpful to administrators who want to compare their facility's performance in specific with a normative group of comparable facilities that have completed the tool.

Thus far, this chapter has discussed the ACCT within the realm of assessment for long-term care facilities. However, the tool also provides the potential for research and the development of an evidence base. Researchers may also be interested in comparing culture change initiatives between facilities and identifying which variables or factors contribute to progress.

The ACCT has the potential for further work, such as assigning weighted points to the prevalence and importance of individual items, which is an area that individuals in the academic community could help develop. It should be noted that although two facilities that complete the tool have the same overall score, they may have two very different foci. The relevance of the sectional scores then becomes critical when building comparisons between facilities and building evidence to showcase where facilities benchmark on specific items. These scores can also help identify how facilities may move through changes within specific areas or categories.

UNDERSTANDING THE CORE PRINCIPLES AND VALUES OF CULTURE CHANGE REFLECTED IN THE ACCT

Many resources established through the Pioneer Network have identified some core values that are paramount in the process of building a culture change paradigm (Misiorski, 2004). These include some of the principles and values illustrated in Table 4.1. They range from understanding the individual resident to creating an environment for change.

TABLE 4.1 Core Values and Principles Measured in the Artifacts of Culture Change Tool

Core Principle	Core Values
Know each person	— Develop a relationship with each resident, knowing his or her needs and wants as well as his or her daily routines — Assign consistent staff to each resident in order to cultivate this relationship
Each person can and does make a difference	— Despite physical or cognitive impairments, every resident can contribute in some way — Find a sense of "purpose" for every resident and offer choices for care routines, dining, and activities
Relationship is the fundamental building block of a transformed culture	— Enhancing the relationships of staff with residents, with each other, and with residents' families can improve the overall quality of life for each resident — Incorporate a "Best Friends" approach to caring for the resident
Respond to spirit, as well as mind and body	— Move from a task-oriented, medical model of care to one that is holistic and all encompassing, addressing the entire well-being of each person
Risk taking is a normal part of life	— Allow the resident to make personal choices even if that choice results in the resident taking a risk

(continued)

TABLE 4.1 Core Values and Principles Measured in the Artifacts of Culture Change Tool (*continued*)

Core Principle	Core Values
Put the person before the task	— Take an approach to caring for each resident that places the priority on the care of the resident and not just on "getting the task done"
All elders are entitled to self-determination, wherever they live	— Once people move into a long-term care setting, they still have the same rights to make personal decisions (regardless of the outcome) as they did when they resided in their own homes
Community is the antidote to institutionalization	— Change the environment from one of little or no choices and no relationships to one of self-determination, "family," and a sincere sense of community
Do unto others as you would have them do unto you	— The staff treat each other, as well as the residents, as they themselves would like to be treated
Promote the growth and development of all	— Shape and use the potential of the environment in all aspects: physical, organizational, and psychosocial/spiritual
Practice self-examination, searching for new creativity and opportunities for doing better	— Recognize that culture change and transformation are not destinations but a journey—always a work in progress

(Adapted from Misiorski, 2004)

KEY AREAS OF CULTURE CHANGE ADDRESSED BY THE ACCT

The ACCT identifies six specific domains within which specific items are delineated with the goal of creating a homelike setting. These domains include the environment, family and community practices, care practices, leadership practices, and workplace practices and outcomes. The chapters in Part II of this book address each of the domains and associated benchmarks in much more detail. Table 4.2 provides a visual outline of these domains.

Embedded throughout the domains of the ACCT are some specific areas for change and development. What follows are focus areas including strategies to illustrate how to transform a long-term care facility from the medical model to a paradigm that reflects culture change.

TABLE 4.2 Domains Addressed Within the Artifacts of Culture Change Tool

Domain	Chapter in This Book That Addresses This Domain
Care practices	Chapter 5
Environment	Chapter 6
Family and community	Chapter 7
Leadership	Chapter 8
Workplace	Chapter 9
Outcomes	Chapter 10

The Environment

The domain that encompasses the environment strives to work toward physical changes in the long-term care setting to make the environment more homelike. Some examples within the ACCT of strategies to facilitate these physical changes include the following:

a. The lobby area is decorated and inviting to residents and their families/visitors.
b. Private rooms are available and occupied by residents.
c. The traditional public announcement system is not operational; instead, staff use cell phones, text messages, and two-way radios to communicate.
d. The individualization and personalization of rooms, such as paint and décor, are obvious and welcoming.
e. The elimination of traditional nursing stations has taken place, and staff work in common spaces for charting and other work-related activities.
f. The bathing areas are made more homelike through painting, installing towel bars, décor, aromatherapy, and spa-type touches.
g. The living space areas are broken into households, with smaller kitchenette areas and common living areas outside the resident's room within pods of up to 12 people.
h. Conditions provide residents the opportunity to have pets in the home.
i. There is increased lighting in individual rooms and common areas.

The Dining Experience

The dining experience is probably one of the most important of all experiences during the day. Some examples of strategies identified within the tool to address this experience include:

a. Elimination of dining trays delivered to each room
b. Buffet style dining, use of steam trays in the dining room
c. Preparing eggs to order (using pasteurized eggs)
d. Offering multiple choices on a daily basis
e. Knowing each resident's daily pleasures for dining and ensuring that preferences are available
f. Providing a choice of time when each resident would like to dine
g. Offering residents the opportunity to eat in between meals at their own discretion, and making snacks available
h. Giving residents the choice of whom they can share their dining time with
i. Ensuring that all staff are interacting and dining with the residents

Resident Choices

Resident choices help promote autonomy and maintain one's dignity. Some of the examples of resident choices that are addressed by the ACCT include:

a. Bathing when and how each resident chooses—not on a schedule determined by staff
b. The elimination of a traditional "med pass" and instead providing residents with their medications in their rooms
c. Embracing the "I-Care Plan," allowing the resident to create his or her own plan of care
d. Including residents in hiring decisions
e. Providing activities that residents choose on the basis of their wishes, likes, and preferences

Staff Empowerment

A significant part of culture change includes the process of empowering staff so that they can act in the best interests of the residents and make decisions accordingly. Some specific strategies to facilitate staff empowerment that are incorporated within the ACCT include:

a. Building a team workplace environment as opposed to a hierarchical model
b. Providing staff with the opportunity for flexibility in decision making, with a focus and priority on the residents' needs and choices
c. Creating the ability for the staff to develop their own schedules
d. Enabling the staff to take the initiative with physicians regarding the reduction or elimination of medications
e. Creating opportunities for staff to interact with residents and to have time for conversation rather than specifically doing a task

Relationship Building

The ACCT facilitates relationship building between staff and residents. The Care Practices domain (Schoeneman & Bowman, 2006) will focus upon these strategies to include the following:

a. Consistent assignments of permanent staff to each resident
b. Changing the way the staff speak to each other and to residents. Eliminating words and phrases such as *feeder*, *nursing home*, *new admit*, *that's not my job* and *toileting*, as well as "CNA" and other acronyms
c. Incorporating "spa assistants" the same staff who consistently provide the bathing care
d. Providing an opportunity for residents to be a host/hostess to visitors, offering a refreshment or a private space for entertaining

Self-Assessment

The ACCT provides a clear-cut opportunity to develop a baseline as well as clear benchmarks that are useful for self-assessment within facilities. This can be accomplished through the following:

a. Assessment of the current environment and care practices on an ongoing basis in order to identify areas of improvement and to measure outcomes
b. Reevaluation of specific practices to identify changes conducted on a regular series of intervals, such as every 3 months or every 6 months.

Potential Outcomes

The use of the ACCT provides for a series of benchmarks within long-term care that will lead to a series of potential outcomes:

  a. Improved overall quality of life for residents
  b. Improved staff morale and job satisfaction
  c. Decreased staff turnover rates
  d. Decreased burnout and potential for compassion fatigue
  e. Increased occupancy
  f. Decreased food costs
  g. Decreased state survey violations
  h. A reduction in behavioral issues with residents
  i. A reduction in the need for psychotropic medications
  j. Documented improvements in the medical and psychological condition of residents

Although this is not an exhaustive list, it does address key areas of improvement that can be documented through the use of the ACCT, which in turn can lead to improvements in care practices within long-term care settings.

SUMMARY

This chapter reviewed the purpose, history, components, future, values, and principles that underlie the ACCT. The chapter also examined the psychometric properties of this instrument to help address issues of validity and reliability. Examples of the types of items the ACCT measures also were addressed. The chapter concludes with a copy of the ACCT.

DISCUSSION/REFLECTION QUESTIONS

1. *Describe the process of development that the architects of the ACCT underwent to develop it.*
2. *Considering your answer in Question 1, what would you do differently to develop a tool, and what steps would you maintain?*
3. *How are the values and principles that underlie the ACCT similar to or different from the principles and values that would be embraced within the medical model paradigm?*

4. Working with a long-term care facility to which you have access, either alone or with a group offer to help assess aspects of the facility using the ACCT. Once this has been completed, what did you learn through this process? What areas do you still need some instruction, or coaching/mentoring to be comfortable with?

ARTIFACTS OF CULTURE CHANGE ASSESSMENT TOOL

Artifacts of Culture Change

Home name _____ Date _____
City _____ State _____ Current number of residents _____

Care Practice Artifacts

1.	Percentage of residents who are offered any of the following styles of dining: • Restaurant style where staff take residents' orders. • Buffet style where residents help themselves or tell staff what they want. • Family style where food is served in bowls on dining tables where residents help themselves or staff assist them. • Open dining where a meal is available for at least a 2 hour time period and residents can come when they choose; • 24-hour dining where residents can order food from the kitchen 24 hours a day.	_____ Enter the actual percentage % in your home Convert your home's figure based on the below scale: 100–81% (5 points) 80–61% (4 points) 60–41% (3 points) 40–21% (2 points) 20–1% (1 point) 0% (0 points)
2.	Snacks/drinks available at all times to all residents at no additional cost, i.e., in a stocked pantry, refrigerator or snack bar.	_____ All residents (5 points) _____ Some residents (3 points) _____ Not a current practice (0 points)

(continued)

Care Practice Artifacts (*continued*)

3.	Baked goods are baked on resident living areas.	_____ Enter the actual number of days in your home Convert your home's figure based on the below scale: All days of the week (5 points) 2–6 d/wk (3 points) <2 d/wk (0 points)
4.	Home celebrates residents' individual birthdays rather than, or in addition to, celebrating resident birthdays in a group each month.	____ All residents (5 points) ____ Some residents (3 points) ____ Not a current practice (0 points)
5.	Home offers aromatherapy to residents by staff or volunteers.	____ All residents (5 points) ____ Some residents (3 points) ____ Not a current practice (0 points)
6.	Home offers massage to residents by staff or volunteers.	____ All residents (5 points) ____ Some residents (3 points) ____ Not a current practice (0 points)
7.	Home has dog(s) and/or cats(s).	____ At least one dog or one cat lives on premises (5 points) ____ The only animals in the building are when staff bring them during work hours (3 points) ____ The only animals in the building are those brought in for special activities or by families (1 point) ____ None (0 points)
8.	Home permits residents to bring own dog and/or cat to live with them in the home.	____ Yes (5 points) ____ No (0 points)
9.	Waking time/bedtimes chosen by residents.	____ All residents (5 points) ____ Some residents (3 points) ____ Not a current practice (0 points)
10.	"Bathing Without a Battle" techniques are used with residents.	____ All residents (5 points) ____ Some residents (3 points) ____ Not a current practice (0 points)
11.	Residents can get a bath/shower as often as they would like.	____ All residents (5 points) ____ Some residents (3 points) ____ Not a current practice (0 points)
12.	Home arranges for someone to be with a dying resident at all times (unless they prefer to be alone) – family, friends, volunteers or staff.	____ All residents (5 points) ____ Some residents (3 points) ____ Not a current practice (0 points)
13.	Memorials/remembrances are held for individual residents upon death.	____ All residents (5 points) ____ Some residents (3 points) ____ Not a current practice (0 points)

14.	"I" format care plans, in the voice of the resident and in the first person, are used.	____ All care plans (5 points) ____ Some (3 points) ____ Not a current practice (0 points)

Care Practice Artifacts Total (Out of 70 Possible Points)

Environment Artifacts

15.	Percent of residents who live in households that are self-contained with full kitchen, living room and dining room.	_____ Enter the actual percentage in your home Convert your home's figure based on the below scale: 100–81% (100 points) 80–61% (80 points) 60–41% (60 points) 40–21% (40 points) 20–1% (20 points) 0% (0 points)
16.	Percent of residents in private rooms.	_____ Enter the actual percentage in your home Convert your home's figure based on the below scale: 100–81% (50 points) 80–61% (40 points) 60–41% (30 points) 40–21% (20 points) 20–1% (10 points) 0% (0 points)
17.	Percent of residents in privacy-enhanced shared rooms where residents can access their own space without trespassing through the other resident's space. (This does not include the traditional privacy curtain.)	_____ Enter the actual percentage in your home Convert your home's figure based on the below scale: 100–81% (25 points) 80–61% (20 points) 60–41% (15 points) 40–21% (10 points) 20–1% (5 points) 0% (0 points)
18.	No traditional nurses' stations or traditional nurses' stations have been removed.	____ No traditional nurses' stations (25 points) ____ Some traditional nurses' stations have been removed (15 points) ____ Traditional nurses' stations remain in place (0 points)

(continued)

Care Practice Artifacts (*continued*)

19.	Percent of residents who have a direct window view not past another resident's bed.	_____ Enter the actual percentage % in your home Convert your home's figure based on the below scale: _____ 100–68% (5 points) _____ 67–34% (3 points) _____ 33–0% (0 points)
20.	Resident bathroom mirrors are wheelchair accessible and/or adjustable in order to be visible to a seated or standing resident.	_____ All resident bathroom mirrors (5 points) _____ Some (3 points) _____ None (0 points)
21.	Sinks in resident bathrooms are wheelchair accessible with clearance below sink for wheelchair.	_____ All resident bathroom sinks (5 points) _____ Some (3 points) _____ None (0 points)
22.	Sinks used by residents have adaptive/easy-to-use lever or paddle handles.	_____ All sinks (5 points) _____ Some (3 points) _____ None (0 points)
23.	Adaptive handles, enhanced for easy use, for doors used by residents (rooms, bathrooms, and public areas).	_____ All resident-used doors (5 points) _____ Some (3 points) _____ None (0 points)
24.	Closets have moveable rods that can be set to different heights.	_____ All closets (5 points) _____ Some (3 points) _____ None (0 points)
25.	Home has no rule prohibiting, and residents are welcome, to decorate their rooms any way they wish including using nails, tape, screws, etc.	_____ Yes (5 points) _____ No (0 points)
26.	Home makes available extra lighting source in resident's room if requested by resident such as floor lamps, reading lamps.	_____ Yes (5 points) _____ No (0 points)
27.	Heat/air conditioning controls can be adjusted in residents' rooms.	_____ All resident rooms (5 points) _____ Some (3 points) _____ None (0 points)
28.	Home provides or invites residents to have their own refrigerators.	_____ Yes (5 points) _____ No (0 points)
29.	Chairs and sofas in public areas have seat heights that vary to comfortably accommodate people of different heights.	_____ Chair seat heights vary by 3" or more (5 points) _____ Chair seat heights vary by less than 3" (3 points) _____ Chair seat heights do not vary (0 points)

30.	Gliders that lock into place when the person rises are available inside the home and/or outside.	_____ Yes (5 points) _____ No (0 points)
31.	Home has store/gift shop/cart available where residents and visitors can purchase gifts, toiletries, snacks, etc.	_____ Yes (5 points) _____ No (0 points)
32.	Residents have regular access to computer/Internet and adaptations are available for independent computer use such as large keyboard or touch screen.	_____ Both Internet access and adaptations (10 points) _____ Access without adaptations (5 points) _____ Neither (0 points)
33.	Workout room available to residents.	_____ Yes (5 points) _____ No (0 points)
34.	Bathing rooms have functional and properly installed heat lamps, radiant heat panels or equivalent.	_____ All bathing rooms (5 points) _____ Some (3 points) _____ None (0 points)
35.	Home warms towels for resident bathing.	_____ All residents (5 points) _____ Some residents (3 points) _____ Not a current practice (0 points)
36.	Accessible, protected outdoor garden/patio provided for independent use by residents. Residents can go in and out independently, including those who use wheelchairs, e.g., residents do not need assistance from staff to open doors or overcome obstacles in traveling to patio.	_____ Available to all residents (5 points) _____ Available for some residents (3 points) _____ Not available (0 points)
37.	Home has outdoor, raised gardens available for resident use.	_____ Available to all residents (5 points) _____ Available for some residents (3 points) _____ Not available (0 points)
38.	Home has outdoor walking/wheeling path that is not a city sidewalk or path.	_____ Available to all residents (5 points) _____ Available for some residents (3 points) _____ Not available (0 points)
39.	Pager/radio/telephone call system is used where residents' calls register on staff's pagers/radios/telephones and staff can use it to communicate with fellow staff.	_____ Yes (5 points) _____ No (0 points)
40.	Overhead paging system has been turned off or is only used in case of emergency.	_____ Yes (5 points) _____ No (0 points)

(continued)

Care Practice Artifacts (*continued*)

41.	Personal clothing is laundered on resident household/neighborhood/unit instead of in a general all-home laundry, and residents/families have access to washer and dryer for own use.	_____ Available to all residents (5 points) _____ Available to some residents (3 points) _____ None (0 points)

Environment Artifacts Total (Out of 320 Possible Points)

Family and Community Artifacts

42.	Regularly scheduled intergenerational program in which children customarily interact with residents.	_____ Weekly (5 points) _____ Monthly or less frequently (3 points) _____ No (0 points)
43.	Home makes space available for community groups to meet in home with residents welcome to attend.	_____ Yes (5 points) _____ Not a current practice (0 points)
44.	Private guestroom available for visitors at no or minimal cost for overnight stays.	_____ Yes (5 points) _____ Not a current practice (0 points)
45.	Home has café/restaurant/tavern/canteen available to residents, families, and visitors at which residents and family can purchase food and drinks daily.	_____ Yes (5 points) _____ No (0 points)
46.	Home has special dining room available for family use/gatherings that excludes regular dining areas.	_____ Yes (5 points) _____ Not a current practice (0 points)
47.	Kitchenette or kitchen area with at least a refrigerator and stove is available to families, residents, and staff where cooking and baking are welcomed.	_____ Yes (5 points) _____ Not a current practice (0 points)

Family and Community Artifacts Total (Out of 30 Possible Points)

Leadership Artifacts

48.	CNAs attend resident care conferences.	_____ All care conferences (5 points) _____ Some (3 points) _____ Not a current practice (0 points)
49.	Residents or family members serve on home quality assessment and assurance (QAA, QI, CQI, QA) committee.	_____ Yes (5 points) _____ Not a current practice (0 points)

50. Residents have an assigned staff member who serves as a "buddy", case coordinator, Guardian Angel, etc., to check with the resident regularly and follow up on any concerns. (This is in addition to an assigned social service staff.)	_____ All new residents (5 points) _____ Some (3 points) _____ Not a current practice (0 points)	
51. Learning Circles or equivalent are used regularly in staff and resident meetings in order to give each person the opportunity to share their opinion/ideas.	_____ Yes (5 points) _____ Not a current practice (0 points)	
52. Community Meetings are held on a regular basis bringing staff, residents and families together as a community.	_____ Yes (5 points) _____ Not a current practice (0 points)	

Leadership Artifacts Total (Out of 25 Possible Points)

Workplace Practice Artifacts

53. RNs consistently work with the residents of the same neighborhood/household/unit (with no rotation).	_____ All RNs (5 points) _____ Some (3 points) _____ Not a current practice (0 points)	
54. LPNs consistently work with the residents of the same neighborhood/household/unit (with no rotation).	_____ All LPNs (5 points) _____ Some (3 points) _____ Not a current practice (0 points)	
55. CNAs consistently work with the residents of the same neighborhood/household/unit (with no rotation).	_____ All CNAs (5 points) _____ Some (3 points) _____ Not a current practice (0 points)	
56. Self-scheduling of work shifts. CNAs develop their own schedule and fill in for absent CNAs. CNAs independently handle the task of scheduling, trading shifts/days, and covering for each other instead of a staffing coordinator.	_____ All CNAs (5 points) _____ Some (3 points) _____ Not a current practice (0 points)	
57. Home pays expenses for non-managerial staff to attend outside conferences/workshops, e.g., CNAs, direct care nurses. Check yes if at least one non-managerial staff member attended an outside conference or workshop paid by the home in past year.	_____ Yes (5 points) _____ Not a current practice (0 points)	

(continued)

Care Practice Artifacts (continued)

58.	Staff is not required to wear uniforms or "scrubs."	_____ Yes (5 points) _____ Not a current practice (0 points)
59.	Percent of other staff cross-trained and certified as CNAs in addition to CNAs in the nursing department.	_____ Enter the actual percentage in your home Convert your home's figure based on the below scale: _____ 100–81 % (5 points) _____ 80–61% (4 points) _____ 60–41% (3 points) _____ 40–21% (2 points) _____ 20–1% (1 point) _____ 0 (0 points)
60.	Activities, informal or formal, are led by staff in other departments such as nursing, housekeeping, or any departments.	_____ Yes (5 points) _____ Not a current practice (0 points)
61.	Awards given to staff to recognize commitment to person-directed care, e.g., Culture Change award, Champion of Change award. This does not include Employee of the Month.	_____ Yes (5 points) _____ Not a current practice (0 points)
62.	Career ladder positions for CNAs, e.g., CNA II, CNA III, team leader, etc. There is a career ladder for CNAs to hold a position higher than base level.	_____ Yes (5 points) _____ Not a current practice (0 points)
63.	Job development programs, e.g., CNA to LPN to RN to NP.	_____ Yes (5 points) _____ Not a current practice (0 points)
64.	Day care onsite available to staff	_____ Yes (5 points) _____ Not a current practice (0 points)
65.	Home has on staff a paid volunteer coordinator in addition to activity director.	_____ Full time (30 hrs/wk or more) (5 points) _____ Part time (15–30 hrs/wk) (3 points) _____ No paid volunteer coordinator (0 points)
66.	Employee evaluations include observable measures of employee support of individual resident choices, control and preferred routines in all aspects of daily living.	_____ All employee evaluations (5 points) _____ Some (3 points) _____ Not a current practice (0 points)

Workplace Practice Artifacts Total (Out of 70 Possible Points)

Staffing Outcomes and Occupancy

67. Average longevity of CNAs (in any position). Add length of employment in years of permanent CNAs and divide by number of CNA staff. _____ Enter your home's average years.	Convert your home's figure based on the below scale: Above 5 years (5 points) 3–5 years (3 points) Below 3 years (0 points)
68. Average longevity of LPNs (in any position). Add length of employment in years of permanent staff LPNs and divide by the number of LPN staff. _____ Enter your home's average years.	Convert your home's figure based on the below scale: Above 5 years (5 points) 3–5 years (3 points) Below 3 years (0 points)
69. Average longevity of RN/GNs (in any position). Add length of employment in years of permanent staff RNs/GNs and divide by the number of RN/GN staff. _____ Enter your home's average years.	Convert your home's figure based on the below scale: Above 5 years (5 points) 3–5 years (3 points) Below 3 years (0 points)
70. Longevity of the Director of Nursing (in any position). _____ Enter your home's figure in years.	Convert your home's figure based on the below scale: Above 5 years (5 points) 3–5 years (3 points) Below 3 years (0 points)
71. Longevity of the Administrator (in any position). _____ Enter your home's figure in years.	Convert your home's figure based on the below scale: Above 5 years (5 points) 3–5 years (3 points) Below 3 years (0 points)
72. Turnover rate for CNAs. Number of CNAs who left, voluntary or involuntary, in previous 12 months divided by the total number of CNAs employed in the previous 12 months. _____ Enter your home's percentage.	Convert your home's figure based on the below scale: 0–19% (5 points) 20–39% (4 points) 40–59% (3 points) 60–79% (2 points) 80–99% (1 point) 100% and above (0 points)

(continued)

Care Practice Artifacts (*continued*)

73. Turnover rate for LPNs. Number of LPNs who left, voluntary or involuntary, in previous 12 months divided by the total number of LPNs employed in the previous 12 months. _____ Enter your home's percentage.	Convert your home's figure based on the below scale: 0–12% (5 points) 13–25% (4 points) 26–38% (3 points) 39–51% (2 points) 52–65% (1 point) 66% and above (0 points)
74. Turnover rate for RNs. Number of RNs who left, voluntary or involuntary, in previous 12 months divided by the total number of RNs employed in the previous 12 months. _____ Enter your home's percentage.	Convert your home's figure based on the below scale: 0–12% (5 points) 13–25% (4 points) 26–38% (3 points) 39–51% (2 points) 52–65% (1 point) 66% and above (0 points)
75. Turnover rate for DONs. _____ Enter number of DONs in the last 12 months	Convert your home's figure based on the below scale: 1 (5 points) 2 (3 points) 3 or more (0 points)
76. Turnover rate for Administrators. _____ Enter number of NHAs in the last 12 months	Convert your home's figure based on the below scale: 1 (5 points) 2 (3 points) 3 or more (0 points)
77. Percent of CNA shifts covered by agency staff over the last month. Total number of CNA shifts (all shifts regardless of hours in a shift) in a 24-hour period; Multiplied by the number of days in the last full month. Of this number, number of shifts covered by an agency CNA. _____ Enter your percentage (agency shifts divided by total number multiplied by days multiplied by 100).	Convert your home's figure based on the below scale: 0% (5 points) 1–5% (3 points) Over 5% (0 points)

78. Percent of nurse shifts covered by agency staff over the last month.	Convert your home's figure based on the below scale:
Total number of nurse shifts (all shifts regardless of hours in a shift) in a 24-hr period.	0% (5 points) 1–5% (3 points) Over 5% (0 points)
Multiplied by the number of days in the last full month.	
Of this number, number of shifts covered by an agency nurse.	
_____ Enter your percentage (agency shifts divided by total number multiplied by days multiplied by 100).	
79. Current occupancy rate.	Convert your home's figure based on the below scale:
_____ Enter your home's occupancy rate	Above average 86–100% (5 points) Average 83–85% (3 points) Below average 0–82% (0 points)

Staffing Outcomes and Occupancy Total (Out of 65 Possible Points)

(Schoeneman & Bowman, 2006)

Figure 4.1 provides on overview for the scoring of the domains within the ACCT.

Artifacts Sections	Potential Points	Score
Care Practices	70	
Environment	320	
Family and Community	30	
Leadership	25	
Workplace Practice	70	
Staffing Outcomes and Occupancy	65	
Artifacts of Culture Change	580	

FIGURE 4.1 Scoring Overview for the ACCT Domains

Source: Developed by the Centers for Medicare and Medicare Services and Edu-Catering, LLP. *ACC-FL adapted with permission.*

REFERENCES

Kane, R. (2001). Long term care and good quality of life: Bringing them closer together. *The Gerontologist, 41,* 292–304.

Kane, R. (2003). Definition, measurement and correlates of quality of life in nursing homes: Toward a reasonable practice, research and policy agenda. *The Gerontologist, 43*(Suppl. 2), 28–36.

Kane, A.R., Pratt, M., Schoeneman, K., Kane, R.L., Bershadsky, B., Cutler, L.J., Giles, K.S., Liu, L., Kang, K., Zhang, L., Kling, K.C., Degenholtz, H.B. (2004). Measures, indicators and improvement of quality of life in nursing homes: Final report. Retrieved March 7, 2012 from http://www.hpm.umn.edu/ltcresourcecenter/research/QOL/Final_Report_to_CMS_Volume_1.pdf

Katz, S. (1970). Progress in development of the index of ADL. *The Gerontologist, 10*(1, Pt. 1), 20–30.

Lawton, M. P. (2001). The physical environment and the person who has Alzheimer's disease. *Aging & Mental Health, 5*(Suppl. 2), 56–64.

Misiorski, S. (2004). Getting Started: A pioneering approach to culture change in long term care organizations. Rochester, NY: The Pioneer Network. p.2.4

Schoeneman, K., & Bowman, C. (2006). *Development of the artifacts of culture change tool: Report of contract HHSM-500-2005-00076P* (Technical report). Baltimore, MD: Centers for Medicaid & Medicare Services. Retrieved from www.artifactsofculturechange.org/Data/Documents/artifacts.pdf

II

Strategies and Benchmarks for Culture Change

The face of communities, at least communities within the developed world, is changing demographically. More people are graying and living longer. Shifts from a nuclear family to situations in which families are more mobile are leaving many frail and elderly family members to the care of long-term settings. These consumers of care, however, have been acclimated to expectations shaped by a consumer-driven society. Thus, expectations will move from being cared for to being a consumer with specific expectations of care—hence the need to shape care settings, especially in long-term facilities.

The chapters in Part II address this challenge and provide an overview of specific benchmarks within six specific content areas as defined by the Artifacts for Culture Change Assessment Tool, developed by the Centers for Medicare & Medicaid. They also outline some specific examples of how these benchmarks have been met through best practice examples and photographic illustrations.

5

Care Practices

Care practices—the way in which care is provided to individuals living in a long-term care setting or nursing home—form the heart and soul of how long-term care facilities deliver support to their residents. These practices form the basis on which many residents and their families define quality or satisfaction. This chapter identifies and examines the care practices identified as benchmarks in the Artifacts for Culture Change Tool (ACCT; Schoeneman & Bowman, 2006), which provide ideas as to how some of these areas can be executed within the culture change paradigm. Examples from facilities that have successfully implemented the care practices identified in the ACCT will be discussed, and illustrations will be presented to provide readers with a visual image of the care practices.

PERSON-CENTERED CARE

The concept of person-centered care (PCC) was first introduced into regulatory expectations for long-term care facilities in 1987 with the passage of the Omnibus Reconciliation Act by Congress. This legislative effort was a direct result of consistent complaints spearheaded by consumers and advocacy groups in the 1980s revolving around substandard care residents received in U.S. nursing homes. The concept of PCC focused on giving the residents more of a say in their preferences and how their lives would be managed on a day-to-day basis (Koren, 2010). The concept of PCC is one that embraces decision making, voice, and choice within care settings that rests with the individual rather than with the professional. The term PCC was coined by British gerontologist Tom Kitwood (1997), who described a philosophy of empowerment that balanced the priorities of work with the priorities of serving the person requiring assistance in nursing facilities. PCC is not organized for staff convenience, efficiency, or other such criteria (Fazio, 2008).

PCC suggests that the approach to providing care to people living in residential settings is very personalized. Within this framework, resident choice is respected and honored (Brune, 2011). Caregivers follow an individualized care plan based on preferences voiced by the resident for care or treatment as opposed to the goals of the system or as defined by a doctor or other professional. This approach is further delineated as care that is based on the person's and/or family's self-identified hopes, aspirations, and goals, which build on the person's and/or family's own assets, interests, and strengths and that is carried out collaboratively with a broadly defined management team responsible for the formal care of the individual (Coleman et al., 2002). PCC encompasses the following dimensions:

- Personhood (e.g., Epp, 2003; Harr & Kasayka, 2000; Kitwood, 1997; Sloane et al., 2004)
- Knowing the person (e.g., Morton, 2000; Talerico, O'Brien, & Swafford, 2003; Shura, Siders, & Dannefer 2011)
- Maximizing choice and autonomy (Mead & Bower, 2000; Ryden, 1992; Williams, 1990)
- Quality care (e.g., Kayser-Jones,1996; Parley, 2001; Rader, Lavelle, Hoeffer, & McKenzie, 1996; Talerico et al., 2003; Werner, Koroknay, Braun, & Cohen-Mansfield, 1994)
- Nurturing relationships (Brooker, 2004; Epp, 2003; Happ, Williams, Strumpf, & Burger, 1996; Swafford, 2003; Williams et al., 1999)
- A supportive physical and organizational environment (e.g., Gould, 2001; Rader & Semradek, 2003; Rantz et al., 2001)

McCormack and McCance (2006), two Irish colleagues, proposed a model for PCC that incorporates these components but adds an essential dimension that includes the development of interpersonal skills between the staff and the individual residents. This can be accomplished by the staff only through a commitment to the job, being clear about one's beliefs and values, and knowing oneself. This introspection benefits residents because their values and beliefs will be identified and honored. The relationship between staff and residents will not be strictly task oriented but built on respect and shared decision making to meet the residents' complete needs, including physical and mental health needs. In their meta-analysis, McCormack and McCance found that outcomes based on a person-centered approach included satisfaction with care, involvement with care, feelings of well-being, and a therapeutic culture. The strongest outcomes were realized in facilities or settings where there were effective staff relationships, supportive organizational systems, power sharing, and the potential for innovation and risk sharing (Kelly, 2007; Kelly & McSweeney, 2009; McCormack & McCance, 2006).

Jones (2011) further built on this definition to suggest that many long-term care facilities are making the transition from an institutional medical model to a PCC model and becoming oriented toward culture change. She suggested that at the core of PCC are the interaction and relationships between the residents and the front-line staff who care for individual residents. This perspective places the onus of responsibility on the front-line care staff, certified nursing assistants, and residential staff, who are traditionally perceived to be at the bottom of the pecking order.

Crandall, White, Schuldheis, and Talerico (2007) define PCC as a key concept that guides initiatives toward the improvement of long-term care settings. Key components of this approach include understanding who the individual resident or person is; giving as many choices as possible and encouraging autonomy; fostering, building, and sustaining relationships; striving for personhood; and facilitating an environment that is supportive of putting the person first (through both the physical and organizational setting). In addition to their definitions of PCC, Crandall and colleagues examined strategies that promote these care practices within facilities, and they found approaches that would help facilities build PCC practices within the organization. These practices include engaging the individual residents, engaging the staff, ensuring that systems within the organization support a PCC practice philosophy, and ensuring that the overall organizational structure can support the sustainability of a PCC approach to care. These are described in greater detail in Part III of this book in an effort to help readers understand how to engage, plan, facilitate, and sustain a person-centered approach to care.

THE LINK AMONG PERSON-CENTERED CARE, AUTONOMY, AND WELL-BEING

Thus far, this chapter has made the case for the role of the actual practice of care and how specific practices will lead to improved quality of life. Hammarstrom and Torres (2012) studied how people "aging in place" viewed quality of life and well-being. They identified well-being through themes of acceptance, predictability, and control. These perspectives can be maintained among older people who are losing cognitive and functional capacities, regardless of socioeconomic conditions or factors, or physical and mental capacity, if some specific elements are in place. Hammarstrom and Torres found that, with acceptance, predictability, and control, there was a direct link among these three elements and positive well-being within nursing home settings. Stewart and her colleagues (2000) examined the impact of PCC on health outcomes in a Canadian setting and found that PCC led to better health outcomes, less discomfort on the part of the consumer, and fewer diagnostic procedures and tests required as part of the medical intervention process.

Up to this point, this chapter has reviewed the concept of PCC practices and discussed their relative importance in care settings. In the next section, a host of care practice benchmarks are described and discussed, and some examples are showcased.

CARE PRACTICE BENCHMARKS

This segment identifies a number of care practice benchmarks that facilities can address in an effort to make their setting more homelike and work within the realm of the culture change paradigm.

Dining

Benchmark: The ACCT benchmark for dining measures the percentage of residents who are offered any of the following styles of dining:

- Restaurant style, where staff take resident orders
- Buffet style, where residents help themselves or tell staff what they want
- Family style, where food is served in bowls on dining tables and residents help themselves or staff assist them
- Open dining, where the meal is available for at least a 2-hour time period and residents can come and eat when they choose
- 24-hour dining, where residents can order food from the kitchen 24 hours a day

The concept of food preferences and weight control have been well documented in the literature (Institute for Caregiver Education, 2006; Rantz & Flesner, 2004; Ronch & Weiner, 2003). Offering people food preferences and choices helps them maintain their weight. Some strategies to facilitate these dining options can include the availability of food and drinks at all times through a "snack bar"–designated area that is open 24 hours per day. In addition, access to the kitchen in the evenings and during the night shift promotes choice for individuals.

A challenge or barrier that many facilities may face is the idea that there will be much food wasted or a lack of control over the food budget if food is consumed at will, especially during the evening (Calkins, Kator, Wyatt, & Halliday, 2009). The reality, however, is that once individual preferences are monitored, it will be easier to be able to identify what people may request and to plan ahead for the availability of these food choices. Ronch and Weiner (2003) found, while studying a facility in Providence, Rhode Island, that less food was, in fact, wasted, because the staff know the individual residents and their personal preferences. Residents had the option of dining within neighborhood kitchen settings. Ronch and Weiner also found that, over a period of 6 years, the number of residents with weight loss issues declined from 20 to three, and they accounted for this as due to the ability to exercise control over food outside of mealtimes.

In a restaurant-style dining option, where staff are responsible for taking resident orders prior to eating, the options to facilitate this process can take several forms. Daily menus can be available with menu choices for residents. Some facilities have two different entrees prepared for residents, and a choice of side dishes (e.g., three vegetable options, and residents may choose one or two vegetable items and one starch item). Residents also have a choice of beverage items. Generally speaking, this option is coordinated with other unit staff members so that the choices are prepared while keeping in mind the residents and their food preferences (Calkins et al., 2009). If a resident is limited in his or her decision-making ability, then a nursing assistant or a family member may help in the food planning options. In some instances, these menu choices are made up to a week ahead of time as a help to dietary planning. When residents are more mobile and higher functioning (e.g., in rehabilitation settings or in an assisted living facility), they may pre-order their meals in an effort to help with the planning but actually order during mealtime. The process of pre-ordering will enable the dietary staff to ensure that the menu item will be available, but the process of confirming the order can help the individual recognize that he or she has requested some specific meal items. This approach allows residents to eat one course at a time and enjoy their food. It also allows the meal to be broken down into different forms, ranging from cutting one's own food, to eating more finely processed foods (when the person no longer has the ability to eat with utensils).

With buffet style dining, where residents help themselves or tell staff what they want, residents may have numerous food choices, to include at least two main entrées, hot side items, and desserts. In addition, a soup and salad bar may be available. In the buffet options, homes may need to invest in a steam table to keep the food warm, and menu options may need to be printed on cards at resident dining tables. The steam table will help keep food warm over a 2-hour period when food is made available to residents at their mealtime. The menu options will enable those with mobility problems to have an aide help choose their meal selection and bring the food back to the dining table. Homes or communities that have restaurants available on site may also set up an option for dining via the buffet, and residents can choose food selections accordingly. Shell Point Village, located in Fort Myers, Florida, exercises this option (personal communication, Rich Cerrina, June 6, 2012). They provide buffet options in at least one of their restaurants for residents and friends/family who may be visiting. Menus are developed and advertised using a monthly calendar for residents within the community. Figures 5.1 and 5.2 provide some illustrations of food buffet dining room layouts. These layouts, which include a steam table, become essential in the development of this choice-based approach.

A third dining option is a family-style approach, in which food is served in bowls on dining tables, and residents help themselves or staff assist them. Some debate about the viability of this option is sometimes questioned because portion control may be of concern. In this option, food portions may be controlled through using serving utensils that are one-half cup in size (4 oz). Residents may feel that this option more closely resembles the dining opportunities that they experienced within their own homes, seated around a table with friends or family members. In addition to the actual appeal of the food, the serving bowls that are used may be brightly colored to create some vitality in the environment.

Dekalb (IL) County Rehabilitation and Nursing Center adopted a family-style dining approach because many of their residents were people who had been raised on a farm, or had a large family, and were used to family-style dining. The facility implemented a practice whereby individuals with weight concerns were weighed once a week in an effort to keep track of changes in body weight due to lack of portion control when using the family-style dining approach. People without a weight problem were weighed monthly (Illinois Pioneer Coalition, 2010).

A fourth dining option is the open-dining approach, where meals are available for at least a 2-hour period and residents can eat when they choose. This option may be more realistic for more mobile residents, who may have set activities during the day. Some facilities, however, experience a situation in which residents look toward mealtimes as an event and are seated within the dining area at least a half-hour prior to mealtimes.

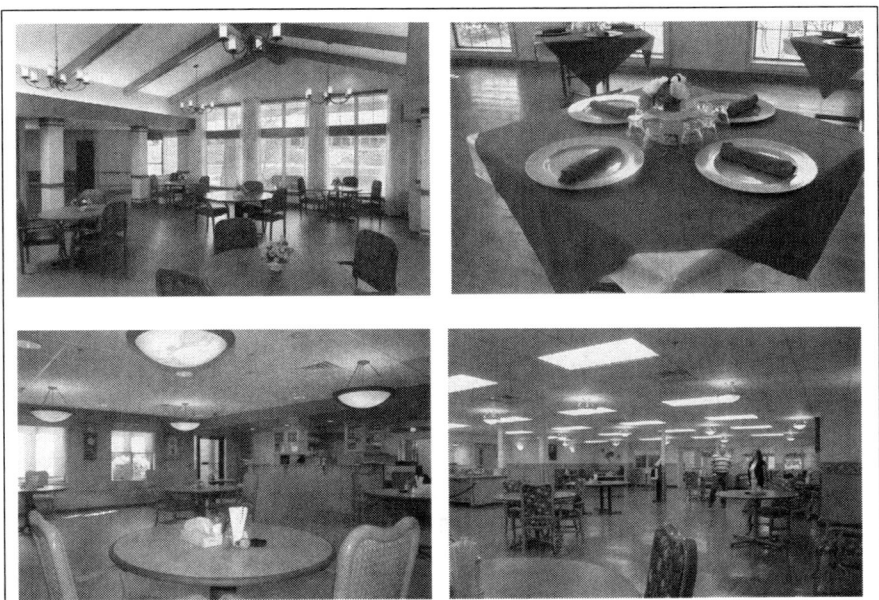

FIGURE 5.1 Dining Option Layouts

Source: Horty Elving Architectural Group. Top right image courtesy of Tuscany Village.

A fifth option includes the opportunity for 24-hour dining, where residents can order food from the kitchen around the clock. On the surface, this approach may seem unrealistic because administrative staff may fear that orders for food will be placed at whim throughout the day. In reality, this concern is unfounded, because people tend to be accustomed to their mealtimes, but they may like to order something at additional times of day. Other people may miss a meal because of outside appointments and would like to be able to order food upon their return or at their convenience. In general, people are creatures of habit, and if this approach is one that fits a person's lifestyle, this behavior will become apparent early or during intake. Once a resident's preferences are known to a facility, the staff can plan for these options. Having food available 24 hours per day may also facilitate some cross-training on the part of aides who may have to double as short-order duty kitchen staff. Figures 5.1 and 5.2 provide different images of dining layouts within long-term care facilities. The first segment of images in Figure 5.1 provides dining layout options, while Figure 5.2 provides options for buffet dining room layouts.

A cooking club is another option available to inspire some variety in the dining experience. Residents can sign up to participate in this type of event, which gives them the opportunity to share their favorite recipes and work with others in the preparation of culinary delights. The staff at

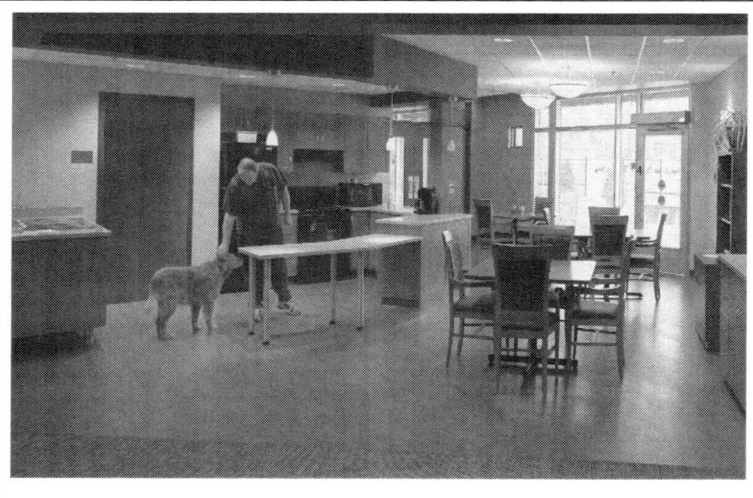

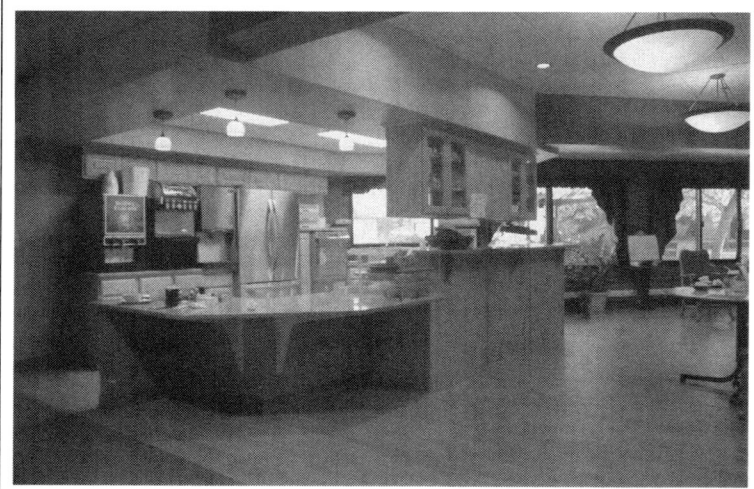

FIGURE 5.2 Buffet Dining Room Layout
Source: Horty Elving Architectural Group

Oak Crest Residence and Atrium Apartments in Elgin, IL, has embraced this concept, and they host a monthly cooking club. Participants choose a weekly menu and recipes. The staff help residents work in small groups to prepare the recipes. Outcomes or benefits from this approach include socialization, laughter, and reminiscence (Illinois Pioneer Coalition, 2010). If this approach is tried, a couple of words of caution are important: First, double or triple the recipe and, second, be mindful that some of the more alert participants may want to dominate the experience!

Snacks/Light Refreshments

> Benchmark: Snacks/drinks are available at all times to all residents at no additional cost; for example, in a stocked pantry, refrigerator, or snack bar.

Snacks can be easily addressed as a benchmark in facilities through identifying a specific area as the "local snack bar" and ensuring that it is stocked on a routine basis. This approach leads to an enhanced home-like culture, when one can easily access the snack bar for food or drink at any time during the day. Bump (2005) suggested that "Food is the heart of the home. . . .The ideal is to have what the residents want to eat available 24 hours a day, 7 days a week with the opportunity to eat with whom they wish, in places they choose to be" (p. 33)

In terms of beverages, "spa" water offers a refreshing touch and provides an ideal way to hydrate residents. Spa water can easily be made by combining cut-up fruits or cut-up cucumber slices with water in a large pitcher. Orange, peach, or strawberry slices combined with ice water provide a wonderful refreshing touch and help with hydration. Slices of lemon or limes in water provide another version of spa water, or sprigs of mint also add a nice touch!

Facilities have handled the option of serving light beverages in a variety of ways. In some cases, a snack corner is available in an area where residents can easily access a soft drink/soda, and a coffee machine is available. Single-serving coffee and tea selections are also available, along with some fresh fruit and fresh cookies. In some cases, a mini-bar is available to residents and refrigerated snacks are available. Aides also provide beverages and host a "happy hour" routinely each afternoon to ensure that people are adequately hydrated, especially with water.

In a study conducted by the Pioneer Network (2011) among facilities that have engaged in culture change through the ACCT (Centers for Medicare and Medicaid, 1997), of 319 respondents, 259 (81.9%) had fully implemented this benchmark.

Baked Goods

> Benchmark: Baked goods are baked within the residents' living areas.

The aroma of baked goods has a positive impact on one's psyche. The Green House Project (2005) found that the aroma of baked goods increased residents' appetites, and they also ate better. Hitz Memorial Home, located in Highland, IL, found that residents were also more engaged in their social activities when they had the opportunity to share recipes and participate in the baking process (Jurkowski, 2011). In the event that it is not possible for a facility to bake cookies or other goods with ingredients from scratch, options for preportioned unbaked goods may help meet this option. Baking on site can still provide the opportunity to create the aroma of fresh baked goods, and the preportioned option helps save the kitchen staff time and energy in the preparation phase, with a similar outcome to fresh baked goods.

In a study conducted by the Pioneer Network (2011), among facilities who have engaged in culture change through the ACCT, of 319 respondents, 221 (69.3%) had not implemented this benchmark at all.

Birthdays

> Benchmark: The facility celebrates residents' individual birthdays rather than, or in addition to, celebrating resident birthdays in a group each month.

The celebration of monthly birthdays acknowledges these events as a group; however, nothing can replace the individualized nature of affirming one's personhood and importance through a personal birthday celebration. If a facility is divided into households, a personal and individualized birthday celebration can take place easily within a neighborhood household. Volunteers such as church groups or school groups could be invited to participate in helping to organize birthday celebrations in an effort to personalize the event and make the celebration a time to remember. Many academic institutions look for service-learning activities with long-term care facilities or community entities to integrate their students into. These collaborations can prove to be a positive venue for helping to facilitate this benchmark.

Creating a space to celebrate birthdays; for families is also an essential component of this benchmark. Figure 5.3 illustrates one option of celebrating birthdays; using a family dining area.

In a study conducted by the Pioneer Network (2011), among facilities that have engaged in culture change through the ACCT, of 319 respondents, 194 (60.8%) had fully implemented this benchmark.

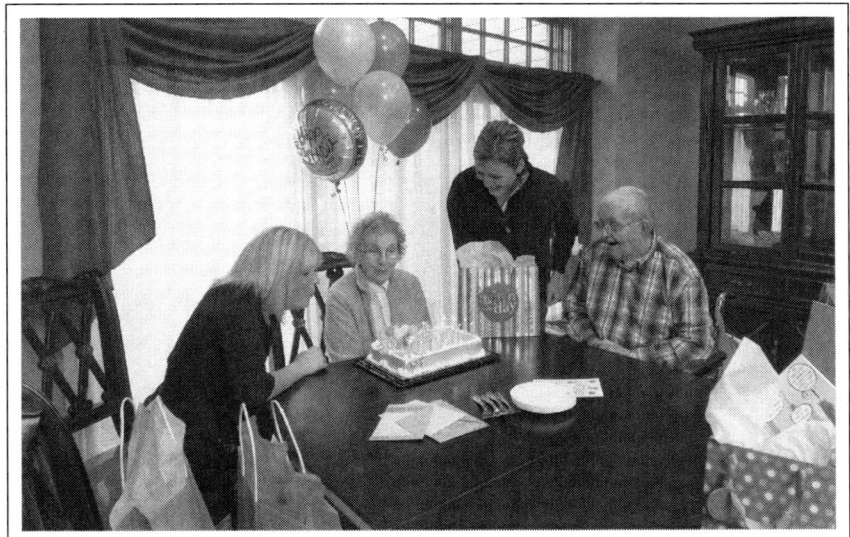

FIGURE 5.3 Birthday Celebration
Source: Horty Elving Architectural Group

Aromatherapy

> Benchmark: The facility offers aromatherapy to residents by staff or volunteers.

In this benchmark, facilities strive to offer aromatherapy to residents by staff or volunteers. Although a relatively new concept, the research literature suggests that there are positive benefits from the use of aromatherapy interventions. The use of aromatherapy has also been found to mask odors associated with care facilities, such as those resulting from incontinence. The literature also suggests that essential oils have an impact on the reduction of anxiety and the improvement of quality of life for cancer patients (Lin, Chan, & Lam, 2007; McBee, Westreich, & Likourezos, 2004), and aromatherapy was found to reduce signs of distress, anxiety, and agitation in residents with Alzheimer's disease (Snyder, Egan, & Burns, 2005). Other impacts of aromatherapy include reduced agitation among people with dementia, improved sleep patterns, and the perception of reduced pain (Kunstler et al., 2004). Additional clinical evidence has reported that the use of essential oils can have a positive impact on one's appetite, sundowning behaviors, short-term memory, and weight loss (Gray & Clair, 2002; Lin et al., 2007; Trombley, Thomas, & Mosher-Ashley, 2003). Clinical evidence has also found that the use of aromatherapy reduces aggressive behavior such as screaming and physical contact with others, along with nonaggressive behaviors, such as pacing and anxiety. (Conn & Seitz, 2010; Snow, 2004; Fitzsimmons, 2002; N.C. Coalition for Long Term Care Enhancement, 2006).

In a study conducted by the Pioneer Network (2011) among facilities that have engaged in culture change through the ACCT, of 319 respondents, 224 (70.2%) had not implemented this benchmark at all.

Massage

Benchmark: The facility offers massage to residents by staff or volunteers.

Hand massage and gentle touch have been found to reduce anxiety in seniors (Cheung 1999; McBee, 2008) and to reduce agitation (Synder et al., 2005). In a clinical trial that examined the effectiveness of massage therapy for nursing home residents, Cheung (1999) observed the outcomes of functioning and activities of daily living with individuals who were seen by both a social worker and a massage therapist. The findings suggested that there were improvements in activities of daily living when the massage therapist worked in combination with the social worker. Corbin, Mellis, Beaty, and Kutner (2009) examined the impacts of massage therapy and other complementary and alternative medicine therapies with patients who had cancer and found that massage therapy reduced pain in patients with advanced cancer.

Once again, opportunities for massage present as an excellent opportunity to utilize volunteers. Beauty specialists such as local Mary Kay consultants are often eager to provide service to the community and "pamper" hands! Readily available in most communities, such consultants work with community service projects, including assisted living and long-term care settings, and they can be part of an initial step in building the gentle effectiveness of hand massage. In addition, a number of strategies that can be useful to caregivers can be found in McBee's (2008) text *Mindfulness-Based Elder Care: A CAM Model for Frail Elders and Their Caregivers.*

In a study conducted by the Pioneer Network (2011) among facilities that have engaged in culture change through the ACCT, of 319 respondents, 227 (71.1%) had not implemented this benchmark at all.

Facility Pets

> Benchmark: The facility has dog(s) and/or cat(s) that are the "facility" pet(s).

Companion animals have been documented in the literature as having multiple benefits for the staff and residents. Earlier studies on quality of life have found a positive correlation between quality of life and numbers of house pets (e.g., Kane et al., 2004). Companion animals have a number of physical benefits for the individual, including lower blood pressure and pulse rate, fewer physician visits, enhanced opportunities for socialization, increased activity, opportunities for affection and unconditional love, increased adaptation to grief and loss, improved attentiveness to one's personal care, decreased levels of depression, fewer headaches, and fewer problems with sleeping (Compas & Gittler, 2009; Giaquinto & Valentini, 2009; Le Roux & Kemp, 2009; Ruckdeschel & Van Haitsma, 2001). A pet therapy intervention with elderly inpatients living in a long-term care setting found that the program was effective in improving both depression and cognitive functioning for residents, especially the oldest-old (80+). Depression symptoms were reduced by at least 50% in the sample, as measured by the Geriatric Depression Inventory, and scores improved on the Mini-Mental Status Examination (Moretti et al., 2010).

Common pets include birds, parrots, cockatiels, and parakeets, which can live in the home's aviary, central to the facility (Coleman et al., 2002; Green House Project, 2005), and promoted through the Eden Alternative. More recently, however, facilities have integrated either a facility dog or cat for residents to pamper, such as the case with a cocker spaniel adopted by Fairview Haven Retirement Community, in Chicago, IL. Middlechurch Home, located in Selkirk, Manitoba, Canada, also boasts of pet goats and rabbits in their facility, which is located in a rural community. The pet goats and rabbits comfort the rural residents, who long to be closer to the animals with which they spent many years during their goat-farming days (Ambrose, B. personal communication, April 9th, 2012).

Despite the benefits to pets, facility staff who are not pet lovers may take offense at having to care for a pet in addition to their daily work. A strategy to help in such cases would be to ask for volunteers to walk, water, and oversee pets during shifts. This may ease the burden for individuals with personal, cultural, or religious preferences against pets in the home.

In a study conducted by the Pioneer Network (2011) among facilities that have engaged in culture change through the ACCT, of 319 respondents, 213 (66.7%) had partially implemented this benchmark.

Resident Pets

> Benchmark: The facility permits residents to bring their own dog and/or cat to live with them in the facility.

Permitting residents to keep their pets when they move into the facility helps them to maintain their autonomy and personal sense of control. Moves are often perceived with a sense of loss and grieving; therefore, any effort to help a transition for residents and enable them to maintain control, including a move with a pet, will make the transition into the residential facility smoother.

Kay, a resident of Aviston Countryside Manor in Aviston, IL, moved into the facility with her pet Chihuahua, Cocoa, who followed her around throughout the facility and spent every waking moment at Kay's side (Illinois Pioneer Coalition, 2010). The daily need for exercise that Cocoa required was instrumental in helping Kay maintain her vitality and mobility. Unfortunately, when Kay passed away early in 2010, her family decided to take Cocoa and provide care for the orphaned pet. However, other residents within the facility missed Cocoa, and after several resident council meetings during which Cocoa's absence was noted, the family agreed to let the facility adopt Cocoa. Thus, residents' pets support not only the individual resident but also many of the resident's neighbors in the facility and provides a multitude of benefits.

The Pioneer Network's benchmark study (2011) among facilities that have engaged in culture change through the ACCT revealed that, of 319 respondents, 267 (83.7%) had partially implemented this benchmark.

Bedtimes

> Benchmark: Waking times/bedtimes are chosen by the residents.

Residents who feel in control of their lives and schedules have been reported to have higher overall morale, better overall functioning in terms of activities of daily living, and lower levels of depression (Martin, Fiorentino, Jouldjian, Josephson, & Alessi, 2010). They have also been reported to be thriving due to circadian rhythms that have been restored (Calkins et al., 2009). Within a culture change environment, residents have the opportunity to define when they prefer to wake and when they would prefer to go to bed. Some individuals prefer to watch television late into the night, whereas others prefer to arise with the sunrise and go to bed with the sunset. The end result of these varying schedules among residents in long-term care settings is that the staff work schedules would have to be developed to accommodate these differences in waking–sleeping schedules. This has traditionally been problematic; however, this goal can be accomplished if the staff have consistent assignments to specific residents (a concept that is defined and developed later in this book).

Scheduling medications can also play a role in one's sleep patterns. In order for facilities to accomplish the goal of residents having uninterrupted sleep cycles, medications need to be given during daytime hours, rather than between 11:00 p.m. to 7:00 a.m. The Lancaster Group (Orland Park, Illinois) made a concerted effort to review each patient's medication regimen with their Medical Officer of Health to determine whether medications were necessary and appropriate for the time administered, if given during the 11:00 p.m. to 7:00 a.m. time frame. Once reviewed, alternatives were sought to administer the medications outside of the overnight time frame (Illinois Pioneer Coalition, 2010). The end result was that residents slept better, with no interruptions; resident problematic behaviors decreased, especially for patients with Alzheimer's disease; and roommates also had better quality of sleep from not being awoken when medication administration to their roommate took place.

Overall, the goal is for facilities and long-term care settings to provide an environment in which residents can enjoy a full 8 hours of sleep without disturbance. In addition, residents should have the opportunity to choose when they would like to retire for the day (rather than competing with a nursing schedule) and when they would like to arise for the day.

In a study conducted by the Pioneer Network (2011) among facilities that have engaged in culture change through the ACCT, of 319 respondents, 172 (53.9%) had partially implemented this benchmark.

Bathing and Bathing Schedules

> Benchmark: "Bathing Without a Battle" techniques are used with residents.

On a typical day in long-term care settings, the bathing experience has been one characterized by an ongoing battle between the resident and staff. Residents, particularly those with dementia, often struggle with being bathed against their will, and behaviors that indicate refusal are largely ignored. The behavior that is ignored moves from overt and sometimes nonverbal refusals to verbal and physical resistance or violence. Sensitivity to the bathing process, and specific strategies to enhance the bathing experience, can lead to a more ideal situation for both resident and caregiver through a more humane approach to bathing.

Since the early 1990s, two research teams have been continuously funded by the National Institutes of Health to develop interventions to improve bathing. In 1997, these two teams were jointly funded to undertake a clinical trial of two interventions in bathing of patients with dementia. In early studies that used these person-centered methods, pre- and postintervention ratings of over 500 videotaped baths found a 56% reduction in aggressive behaviors against caregivers, a 62% reduction in care recipient agitation, a 67% reduction in care recipient distress, and a 38% decrease in the proportion of bathtime spent crying or screaming (Rader et al., 2002; Barrick et al, 2008). Rader and colleagues (2002) found that when the bath and bathing care routines were individualized, a person engaged in less aggressive behaviors. The "Bathing Without a Battle" has been successfully implemented nationwide to help with reducing aggression among patients with dementia in long-term care settings, especially since 2002 when Rader and colleagues published the *Bathing Without a Battle* manual, a resource that offers a step-by-step guide on how to handle the challenges of bathing and provides a program to assist staff and residents with the bathing process.

Some of the equipment and strategies that are incorporated into the bathing process as discussed in Rader et al.'s (2002) manual include grab bars, towel warmers, tub transfer seats, specialized spa tubs and chairs, and specialized bathing products. These products, along with a person-centered strategy to bathing, can shift the bathing experience from one of frustration to one of enjoyment and comfort.

In a study conducted by the Pioneer Network (2011) among facilities that have engaged in culture change through the ACCT, of 319 respondents, 118 (36.9%) had partially implemented this benchmark.

Bathing/Shower Schedules

Benchmark: Residents can get a bath/shower as often as they would like.

Traditionally, bathing and showering schedules have been set around staffing patterns and activity-worker schedules. This approach tends to change the bathing experience from being a valued and an enjoyable event and does not also fit into the person's natural routine that may have been established before he or she entered the facility. Within a culture change approach, residents have the opportunity to bathe and shower when they would like and as often as they would like. For some, this may be in the early morning, but for others it may be another time of day that is convenient. Chung (2010) found that nursing assistants perceived that respect for the individual's dignity and values around bathing care helped promote their personhood and preserve their identity.

Two specific facilities, Wellstar Paulding Nursing Center, in Dallas, GA, and Quality Partners, in Providence, RI, have devised practices whereby people can decide how often, what time of day, and via what method they would like to bathe. Towel warmers also help to shelter the person from the cold after a shower. In some cases, the towel warmers have been found to encourage baths/showers among residents (Illinois Pioneer Coalition, 2010).

In a study conducted by the Pioneer Network (2011), among facilities that have engaged in culture change through the ACCT, of 319 respondents, 213 (66.7%) had partially implemented this benchmark.

Supporting People During Their Last Journey in Life

> Benchmark: The facility arranges for someone—family, friends, volunteers, or staff—to be with a dying resident at all times (unless the individual prefers to be alone).

The process of death and dying can be one that offers grace and speaks to the importance of the journey, or it can be negated altogether. Neglecting the importance of the journey through one's last days can be a tremendous lost opportunity for both the dying individual and the facility. People have a need to share their feelings and honor those with whom they have lived and to whom they have grown close. Opportunities for hospice care in long-term care facilities have been developing at an increasing rate and, along with these programs, the opportunity to allow closure for friends, family, residents, and staff becomes of paramount importance (Berndt, 2004; Illinois Pioneer Coalition, 2010). This area appears to be one well developed in practice, and this may be because facilities tend to consider that long-term care settings may be the last home within a person's life journey.

A variety of practices have been incorporated into various facilities to support people during their last journey in life. Some specific practices that facilities can promote to help with the journey include the following:

- The development of a photo wall to honor and recognize those who have passed on.
- The development of an interdisciplinary work group to develop new practices.
- The building of a task force with residents to design a plan for residents/staff and others to sit with residents who have no family available.
- Using a symbol (e.g., an angel magnet) to signify residents who are receiving comfort care or hospice care. This approach enables an entire team to provide better care due to heightened sensitivity.
- A screen that could be set up in front of a resident's bed so that people walking up and down a hallway would not notice the person who has passed, and family could remain with their loved one with some degree of privacy.
- The creation of a hospitality cart with food and toiletries available to families who are staying long periods of time with dying residents.
- The development of a memorial room where dying residents and their families can stay around the clock. The room would be equipped with a sleeping area and private bathroom and could also be personalized to memorialize the journey. The room could be a project developed through either memorial donations or a fundraising effort.
- Enabling residents to develop and participate in a personalized memorial service or ceremony within the facility as a way of helping them draw closure to the loss of a person within their community (Illinois Pioneer Coalition, 2010; The Chrysalis Project, 2011).

In a study conducted by the Pioneer Network (2011) among facilities that have engaged in culture change through the ACCT, of 319 respondents, 102 (31.9%) had partially implemented this benchmark.

Memorials

> Benchmark: Memorials/remembrances are held for individual residents upon death.

The opportunity for residents to be able to share their experiences with their peers can be powerful in many ways. The process can help bring closure, can help with feelings of grief and loss, sensitize others to the meaning of the loss, and build a bridge between people living within a facility. More important, these care practices help to value life through the dignity of one's death or passing.

Misercordia Place, located in Winnipeg, Manitoba, Canada, offers a memorial service on an annual basis and invites residents' family members, friends, and staff to attend. Each family is asked to prepare a short eulogy or talk about their loved one's legacy in their lives, and residents are given the same opportunity through a resident spokesperson. After sharing stories, a family member representing the bereaved places a rose in a vase to signify that their loved one has departed. The ceremony concludes with some songs and prayer, followed by light refreshments and fellowship for all in a community meeting room (Styles, J. personal communication, July 5, 2012).

The Eden Garden, located in Creve Coeur, MO, offers a monthly memorial service following the passing of residents. This service offers a time for the residents and staff to share their thoughts and feelings about the recently departed, and honors their passing. The service is primarily for the residents and staff.

The Veterans Nursing Home, located in Marion, IL, offers a special memorial service for its veterans upon their passing. Residents and family members gather in the nursing home chapel around an American flag situated next to a photo and/or photo collage of the departed. Once again, stories are shared and people are given the opportunity to find closure with the deceased resident.

Person-First Care Plans

> Benchmark: "I"-format care plans, in the voice of the resident and in the first person, are used.

The use of the first person in personal care planning helps customize the process and enables each resident to be seen as a person first.

Research has found that utilizing "I"-first language helps connect with the individual and creates a personal relationship. All too often, the care plans are written in third-person format, thus impersonalizing the resident. The beauty of person-first language is that the individual is then seen within an active relationship among the interdisciplinary support team. This concept is somewhat novel within the realm of long-term care settings, but it has been utilized within the disability arena for years within individualized care plans (O'Brien & O'Brien, 2002). This approach tends to also help the individual preserve some of his or her personal dignity and autonomy.

SUMMARY

This chapter addressed strategies and benchmarks to enhance the care extended to residents and to create a person-centered approach to long-term care settings. The chapter began with a review of the value of a person-centered approach to care and its impact on an individual's functioning and adaptation. Throughout the chapter, benchmarks to be met in an effort to meet a culture change paradigm within long-term care settings were reviewed, and strategies to address these benchmarks were presented.

DISCUSSION/REFLECTION QUESTIONS

1. *Identify five benchmark areas discussed within this chapter that you would not have thought of in your effort to create care practices more in line with a culture change paradigm.*
2. *Identify five benchmarks within the care practice domain that you feel have been met within facilities that you either worked in or have been exposed to. Explain why you feel these benchmarks were met.*
3. *Identify three strategies that you and your team could use to address at least one (or up to three) specific benchmarks in the care practice domain?*
4. *Think about a service learning project you and your classmates or colleagues could get involved in to help a local facility (or the facility in which you currently work) to help meet one of the benchmarks in the care practice domain. What steps will you need to put into place to accomplish this goal?*

REFERENCES

Barrick, A. L., Rader, J., Hoeffer, B., Sloane, P., Biddle, S. (2008). *Bathing without a battle: Personal Care of Individuals with Dementia.* NY: New York. Springer Publishing Company.

Berndt, J. (2004). *The sanctity of life and the sacredness of death: A journey of putting pioneer values into practice.* Rochester, NY: The Pioneer Network.

Brooker, D. (2004). What is person-centered care in dementia? *Reviews in Clinical Gerontology, 13,* 215–222.

Brune, K. (2011). Culture change in long term care services: Eden-greenhouse-aging in the community. *Educational Gerontology, 37*(6), 506–525. doi:10.1080/03601277.2011.570206

Bump, L. (2005). The process of physical design: Combating homelessness in long-term care. *Culture Change Now, 3,* 10–17.

Calkins, M., Kator, M., Wyatt, A., & Halliday, L. (2009). Culture change in action: Changing the experiential environment. *Long-Term Living: For the Continuing Care Professional, 58*(11), 16.

Centers for Medicare and Medicaid. (1997). Artifacts of Culture Change Tool. Retrieved from: (www.artifactsofculturechange.org)

Cheung, K. M. (1999). Effectiveness of social work treatment and massage therapy for nursing home clients. *Research on Social Work Practice, 9*(2), 229–247.

Chung, G. (2010). Quality of care in nursing homes from the perspective of nursing assistants. *Dissertation Abstracts International Section A: Humanities and Social Sciences, 70*(11-A), 4453.

The Chrysalis Project: An exploration of one's last journey. (2011, August). Interactive presentation given at the annual 11th national conference of the Pioneer Network, St. Louis, MO.

Coleman, M. T., Looney, S., O'Brien, J., Ziegler, C., Pastorino, C. A., & Turner, C. (2002). The Eden Alternative: Findings after 1 year of implementation. *Journals of Gerontology: Series A: Biological Sciences and Medical Sciences, 57,* 422–427.

Compas, C., & Gittler, J. (2009, August). *Culture change for the aging and companion animals in nursing homes: Benefits, risk, barriers, and best practices..* Paper presented at the 9th national conference of the Pioneer Network, Little Rock, AR.

Conn, D. K., & Seitz, D. P. (2010). Advances in the treatment of psychiatric disorders in long term homes. *Current Opinion in Psychiatry, 23*(6), 516–521.

Corbin, L. W., Mellis, B. K., Beaty, B., & Kutner, J. S. (2009). The use of complementary and alternative medicine therapies by patients with advanced cancer and pain in hospice setting: A multicentered, descriptive study. *Journal of Palliative Medicine, 12*(1), 7–8.

Crandall, L. G., White, D. L., Schuldheis, S., & Talerico, K. A. (2007). Initiating person-centered care practices in long-term care facilities. *Journal of Gerontological Nursing, 33*(11), 47–56.

Epp, T. D. (2003). Person-centered dementia care: A vision to be refined. *The Canadian Alzheimer Disease Review 5*(3), 14–19.

Fazio, S. (2008). Person-centered care in residential settings: Taking a look back while continuing to move forward. *Alzheimer's Care Today, 9*(2), 155–161.

Fitzsimmons, S. (2002). Alternative therapies. *American Journal of Alzheimer's Disease and other Dementias, 17*(4)., 200.
Giaquinto, S., & Valentini, F. (2009). Is there a scientific basis for pet therapy? *Disability and Rehabilitation, 31*(7), 595–598.
Gould, M. O. (2001). Resident-centered care: Teresian House takes a team-based approach to care of the elderly. *Health Progress, 82*(6), 56–58.
Gray, S. G., & Clair, A. A. (2002). Influence of aromatherapy on medication administration to restricted care residents with dementia and behavioral challenges. *American Journal of Alzheimer's Disease and other dementias. 17*(3). 169–174.
Green House Project DVD (2005). Retrieved from: http://blog.thegreenhouseproject.org/wp-content/uploads/2011/04/The-Green-House-Project_-Consumer-Toolkit_rev3.pdf. Retrieved March 1, 2013.
Hammarstrom, G. & Torres, S. (2012). Variations of subjective well-being when "aging in place – A matter of acceptance, predictability and control. *Journal of Aging studies. 26.* 192–203.
Happ, M. B., Williams, C. C., Strumpf, N. E., & Burger, S. G. (1996). Individualized care for frail elders: Theory and practice. *Journal of Gerontological Nursing, 22*(3), 7–14.
Harr, R. G., & Kasayka, R. E. (2000). Person-centered dementia care. *Assisted Living Today, 7,* 41–44.
Illinois Pioneer Coalition. (2010). *Tales from the prairie: Culture change practices in Illinois long term care communities.* Quincy, IL: Author.
Institute for Caregiver Education Newsletter. (Spring, 2006)
Jones, C. S. (2011). Person-centered care: The heart of culture change. *Journal of Gerontological Nursing, 37*(6), 18–23. doi:10.3928/00989134-20110302-04
Jurkowski, E. T. (2011). Field trip to Hitz Memorial Nursing Home. December 4th.
Kayser-Jones, J. (1996). Mealtime in nursing homes: The importance of individualized care. *Journal of Gerontological Nursing, 22*(3), 26–31.
Kane, R. A., Bershadsky, B., Degenholta, H., & Liu, J. (2004). Measures, indicators, and improvement of quality of life in nursing homes: Final report. Submitted to Centers for Medicare and Medicaid services.
Kelly, J. (2007). Barriers to achieving patient-centered care in Ireland. *Dimensions of Critical Care Nursing, 26*(1), 29–34.
Kelly, M., & McSweeney, E. (2009). Re-visioning respite: A culture change initiative in a long-term care setting in Eire. *Quality in Ageing, 10*(3), 4–11.
Kitwood, T. (1997). *Dementia reconsidered: The person comes first.* Buckingham, UK: Open University Press.
Koren, M. J. (2010). Person-centered care for nursing home residents: The culture-change movement. *Health Affairs, 29,* 312–317.
Kunstler, R., Greenblatt, F., Moreno, N. (2004). Aromatherapy and hand massage: Therapeutic recreation interventions for pain management. *Therapeutic Recreation Journal, 38*(2), 133–147.
Le Roux, M. C., & Kemp, R. (2009). Effect of a companion dog on depression and anxiety levels of elderly residents in a long-term care facility. *Psychogeriatrics, 9,* 23–26. doi:10.1111/j.1479-8301.2009.00268.x
Lin, P. W., Chan, W. C., & Lam, L. C. (2007). Efficacy of aromatherapy (*Lavandula angustifolia*) as an intervention for agitated behaviours in Chinese older persons with dementia: A cross-over randomized trial. *International Journal of Geriatric Psychiatry, 22,* 405–410.

Martin, J. L., Fiorentino, L., Jouldjian, S., Alessi, C. A. (2010). Sleep quality in resident of assisted living facilities: Effect on quality of life, functional status, and depression. *Journal of the American Geriatrics Society 58*(5), 829–836. DOI: 10.1111/j.1532-5415.2010.02815.x

McBee, L. (2008). *Mindfulness-based elder care: A CAM model for frail elders and their caregivers.* New York, NY: Springer Publishing.

McBee, L., Westreich, L., & Likourezos, A. (2004). A psychoeducational relaxation group for pain and stress management in the nursing home. *Journal of Social Work and Long Term Care, 3*(1), 15–28.

McCormack, B., McCance, T. V. (2006). The person centered nursing conceptual framework. *Journal of Clinical Nursing, 56,* 1–8.

Mead, N., & Bower, P. (2000). Patient centeredness: A conceptual framework and review of the empirical literature. *Social Science & Medicine, 51,* 1087–1110.

Moretti, F., Bernabei, V., Marchetti, L., Forlani, C., DeRonchi, D., & Atti, A. R. (2010). A pet therapy intervention on elderly inpatients: An epidemiological study. *European Psychiatry, 25*(Suppl.), 577.

Morton, I. (2000). Just what is person-centered dementia care? *Journal of Dementia Care, 8*(3), 28–29.

N.C. Coalition for Long Term Care Enhancement. (2006). The influence of aromatherapy on the biological and behavioral markers of individuals with Alzheimer's disease. Spring-Summer, 3–5.

O'Brien, C. L., & O'Brien, J. (2002). The origins of person-centered planning: A community of practice perspective. In S. Holburn & P. M. Vietze (Eds.), *Person-centered planning: Research, practice, and future directions* (pp. 3–37). Baltimore, MD: Paul H. Brookes.

Parley, F. F. (2001). Person-centered outcomes: Are outcomes improved where a person-centered care model is used? *Journal of Learning Disabilities, 5,* 299–308.

Pioneer Network. (2011). *Tools for change summary report.* Retrieved from www.artifactsofculturechange.org/Data/Documents/Tools%20for%20Change-Artifacts%20v3.pdf

Rader, J., Barrick, A., Hoeffer, B., & Sloane, P. (2002). *Bathing without a battle: Personal care of individuals with dementia.* New York. NY: Springer Publishing Company.

Rader, J., Lavelle, M., Hoeffer, B., & McKenzie, D. (1996). Maintaining cleanliness: An individualized approach. *Journal of Gerontological Nursing, 22*(3), 32–38.

Rader, J., & Semradek, J. (2003). Organizational culture and bathing practice: Ending the battle in one facility. *Journal of Social Work in Long-Term Care, 2,* 269–284.

Rantz, M. J. (2003). Does good quality care in nursing homes cost more or less than poor quality care? *Nursing Outlook, 51,* 93–94.

Rantz, M. J., & Flesner, M. K. (2004). *Person centered-care: A model for nursing homes.* Silver Spring, MD: American Nurses Association.

Rantz, M. J., Popejoy, L. L., Petroski, G. F., Madsen, R. W., Mehr, D. R., Zwygart-Stauffacher, M., ... Maas, M. (2001). Randomized clinical trial of a quality improvement intervention in nursing homes. *The Gerontologist, 41,* 525–538.

Ronch, J., & Weiner, A. (2003). *Culture change in long term care.* Binghamton, NY: Haworth Press.

Ruckdeschel, K., & Van Haitsma, K. (2001). The impact of live-in animals and plants on nursing home residents: A pilot longitudinal investigation. *Alzheimer's Care Quarterly, 2*(4), 17–27.

Ryden, M. B. (1992). Alternatives to restraints and psychotropics in the care of aggressive, cognitively impaired elderly persons. In K. C. Buckwalter (Ed.), *Geriatric mental health nursing: Current and future challenges* (pp. 84–93). Thorofare, NJ: Slack.

Schoeneman, K., & Bowman, C. (2006). *Development of the artifacts of culture change tool: Report of contract HHSM-500-2005-00076P* (Technical report). Baltimore, MD: Centers for Medicaid & Medicare Services. Retrieved from www.artifactsofculturechange.org/Data/Documents/artifacts.pdf

Shura, F., Siders, R. A., & Dannefer, D. (2011). Culture change in long-term care: Participatory action research and the role of the resident. *The Gerontologist, 51*(2), 212–225.

Sloane, P. D., Hoeffer, B., Mitchell, C. M., McKenzie, D. A., Barrick, A. L., Rader, J., Koch, G. G. (2004). Effect of person-centered showering and the towel bath on bathing-associated aggression, agitation, and discomfort in nursing home residents with dementia: A randomized controlled trial. *Journal of the American Geriatrics Society, 52*, 1795–1804.

Snow, A. L., Hovanec, L., & Brandt, J. (2004). A controlled trial of aromatherapy for agitation in nursing home patients with dementia. *Journal of Alternative and Complementary Medicine, 10*(3), 431–437.

Stewart, M., Brown, J. B., Donner, A., McWhinney, I., Oates, J., Westen, W. W., & Jordan, J. (2000). The impact of patient-centered care outcomes. *Journal of Family Practice, 49.* 796–804.

Snyder, M., Egan, E. C., & Burns, K. R. (2005). Interventions for decreasing agitation behaviors in persons with dementia. *Journal of Gerontological Nursing. 21* (7). 34–40.

Swafford, K. (2003). *In search of individualized care: A concept analysis.* Unpublished manuscript, Oregon Health & Science University, Portland.

Talerico, K. A., O'Brien, J. A., & Swafford, K. L. (2003). Person-centered care: An important approach for 21st century health care. *Journal of Psychosocial Nursing and Mental Health Services, 41*(11), 12–16.

Trombley, J., Thomas, B., & Mosher-Ashley, P. M. (2003). Massage therapy for elders with Alzheimer's Disease. *Nursing Homes 52*(10). 82–92.

Werner, P., Koroknay, V., Braun, J., & Cohen-Mansfield, J. (1994). Individualized care alternatives used in the process of removing physical restraints in the nursing home. *Journal of the American Geriatrics Society, 42*, 321–325.

Williams, B., Cattell, D., Greenwood, M., LeFevre, S., Murray, I., & Thomas, P. (1999). Exploring "person-centredness": User perspectives on a model of social psychiatry. *Health and Social Care in the Community, 7*, 475–482.

Williams, C. C. (1990). Long-term care and the human spirit. *Generations, 14* (4), 25–29.

6

Environment Benchmarks/ Artifacts

Environmental practices pave the way for how a particular paradigm is exercised within facilities. This book has reviewed the history of long-term care facilities and found that the alignment between such facilities and hospitals paved the way for an institutional approach to long-term care that is shaped by a medical model paradigm. Benchmarks within the environmental arena would need to radically depart from this approach in order to be aligned with a culture change paradigm. Environmental practices form the basis on which many residents and their family define their residence as a home. In this chapter, the environmental practices identified as benchmarks in the Artifacts of Culture Change Tool (ACCT; Schoeneman & Bowman, 2006) are examined and discussed to provide ideas as to how some of these areas can be executed within the culture change paradigm. Examples from successful facilities are provided, and illustrations are presented to provide readers with a visual image of the care practice being discussed.

WHY ARE ENVIRONMENTAL PRACTICES IMPORTANT?

Environmental practices can make the difference between whether people are functioning or not functioning. Lawton (1990) studied the relationship among environment, functioning, and well-being for at least two decades and argued that, by learning to apply choice and self-direction in the everyday uses of their own housing, occupants with any level of intactness or impairment can actively affect their overall quality of life. Rehabilitation experts and advocates of the independent living paradigm maintain that people with functional impairments can navigate and minimize their "disability" with proper environmental supports (Howard, Nieuwenhuijsen, & Saleeby, 2008; Saleeby, 2007). Here is a simple example: A wheelchair-accessible ramp rather than just the availability of stairs can make the difference between a wheelchair-bound person getting into his or her home or not. Environmental practices create a living space, facilitate a least restrictive environment, and make the difference between a facility being perceived as an institution or a home-like environment (Cutler, 2004; Lawton, Fulcomer, & Kleban, 1984).

Lawton and Nahemow (1973) developed an ecological model that has provided a theoretical background for understanding environmental practices through an ecological perspective. This model suggests that functional behavior is a result of the interaction between one's sense of identity and one's adaptation to the environment. Environmental behavior is the outcome of an individual's functional ability to interact with the challenges or demands placed on him or her by the environment. Highly competent people can function in environments that are not very supportive of their limitations, whereas less competent people function at a diminished capacity (Kahana, 1975). One's environment can work to make some functions impossible while encouraging other functions. Ideally, professionals in the field of long-term care want to work toward building an environment that matches a person's ability. To illustrate this point, consider the case of a wheelchair-bound person who is completely capable of getting into a closet and choosing an outfit for the day but cannot reach the clothing rod. That person's functional ability and the environment are not in sync (Kane, 2003).

The physical environment within long-term care settings can neglect to place demands upon the resident, which can result in negative behaviors, boredom, and anxiety, as well as sensory learned helplessness (Langer & Rodin, 1976; Maier & Seligman, 1976). Learned helplessness can result when a person perceives that he or she is not able to control his or her life, or easily carry out his or her wishes or desires. This learned helplessness, along with an environment that challenges a person's functional capacity, can either raise one's competence or functional ability or lead to inactivity and apathy. Ideally, the goal should be to create an environment that challenges one's ability to problem solve and identify new strategies to meet one's functional needs.

THE LINK BETWEEN ENVIRONMENT AND WELL-BEING

The literature is filled with studies that address quality of life issues and tie these issues to one's environment (Baumeister & Tice, 1985; Cutler, 2000; Kaplan, 1983; Karls & Wandrei, 1992). Factors and variables such as color, image, lighting, and space all play roles in the link between environment and well-being (Cutler & Kane, 2004). The importance of the cultural environment has been ignored in the medical model of nursing homes but is gaining more status as nursing homes move toward person-oriented care (Calkins, Kator, Wyatt, & Halliday, 2009; Robinson & Rosher, 2006). Traditions, values, norms, and symbols are part of the cultural environment, as is the emphasis on residential-like settings in long-term care facilities. These categories, whether thought of individually or collectively, affect the quality of life of the residents, staff members, visitors, and volunteers (Cutler, 2007).

Cutler and Kane (2004) further outlined the role that the physical environment plays in the lives of residents in long-term care settings. They suggested that it is useful to categorize the individual characteristics found in the environment into four separate categories: (a) physical, (b) social, (c) psychological, and (d) cultural. Characteristics of the physical environment, such as door width, corridor length, accessible closet rods, sink clearance, and chair height, affect the physical functioning of the user. Characteristics of the psychological environment are individual and more difficult to measure; they include items that evoke memories and images of the past, as well as promote sensory stimuli. These items may comprise not only features supplied by the family but also items brought by the residents themselves, such as family photographs, personal items, and mementoes from their lives. The social environment refers to the interaction of residents in their environment. Privacy, communal dining, and activity spaces all contribute to the social environment.

ENVIRONMENTAL BENCHMARKS

In addition to the care practice benchmarks that were discussed in Chapter 5, a second component of the ACCT addresses environmental benchmarks. The benchmarks are designed to help facilities identify ways in which they can renegotiate their spaces and décor. Larger facilities may face more challenges with the implementation of these benchmarks compared with smaller facilities. Nonetheless, these are probably the practices that would require the most creativity, because they can often involve structure and physical changes.

Self-Contained Household Units

> Benchmark: Percentage of residents who live in households that are self-contained with full kitchen, living room and dining room.

The household model strives to create a natural "family life setting" within a larger facility. The household generally comprises no more than 12 residents, which automatically provides the opportunity to have more say and voice in one's situation. Within this model, staff tools and supplies are decentralized, which enables the staff to provide more efficient care; also, staff within the household pods are cross-trained and generally work with the same residents. Within this household model it also is easier for staff to facilitate resident preferences and choices related to their activities and meals. The smaller size of the units (i.e., 12 or less) also makes it easier to be able to engage all residents in group planning, special events and cooking and preparation of snacks.

Within this model, all cooking, laundry, and general living space takes place in the individual units. The smaller community of residents provides an opportunity for more centralized care and activities. The physical design of the household model includes all the same features one would find in a traditional household: stove, refrigerator, oven, microwave, dishwasher, sink, utensils and cupboards, and laundry facilities. The household model also takes on the components of a household approach. For example, within households, a front door and kitchen are key features. Other key features include some specific dimensions of privacy and a specific culture and décor. The very personal nature of the household approach enables décor that lends itself to a personal touch. Cutler and Kane (2004) recommended that facilities seek materials and furnishings through home improvement stores and discount stores, rather than going to more expensive hospital supply companies. They also recommended that facilities create a gift registry at a local Target or similar inexpensive department store. Often, family members or local service organizations are in search of items to contribute to long-term care homes. Through a gift registry program, facilities may receive a number of appliances or other items that they may not necessarily be able to afford (Cutler & Kane, 2004).

Another approach to creating a household is to get the community at large involved. Local churches have been known to sponsor guest rooms in homeless shelters, so extending this idea into the long-term care facility could be a vital option to help create a household. A local service club or church group could "adopt" a household unit as a service project. The group would then engage in fund-raising efforts to enable them to purchase either furnishings or amenities for specific household units. If there is more than one household unit in a facility, the art of gentle competition between service clubs can also help with the overall outcome.

Staff are responsible for doing resident laundry and, within this type of setting, residents can probably avoid labeling their clothing, because the unit is small enough that specific laundry days can be established for residents. Bowman (2008) found that laundry facilities within households led to fewer misplaced clothes and fewer clothes lost due to shrinkage. Family members are also more likely to wash their loved one's clothes within the household model, which cuts down on work for the nursing and household staff (Bowman, 2008).

A hallmark of many nursing homes is often the nurse's station. Within the household model, the traditional nurse's station is practically eliminated. Medications and charting no longer are carried out within the unit, in the "nurse's space," but rather at a household table, or a work desk. Medications are often locked up in a cabinet or cupboard, instead of on a traditional medication cart (Bowman, 2008).

Some examples of facilities that operate with a household model include Teresian House, located in Albany, NY; Meadowlark Hills, located in Manhattan, KS; Big Fork Valley, in Billings, MT; Evergreen Retirement Community, in Cincinnati, OH; Hitz Home, in Alhambra, IL; and Fairport Baptist Home, located in Fairport, NY. Figure 6.1 provides a glimpse of a kitchen where the household model is in place.

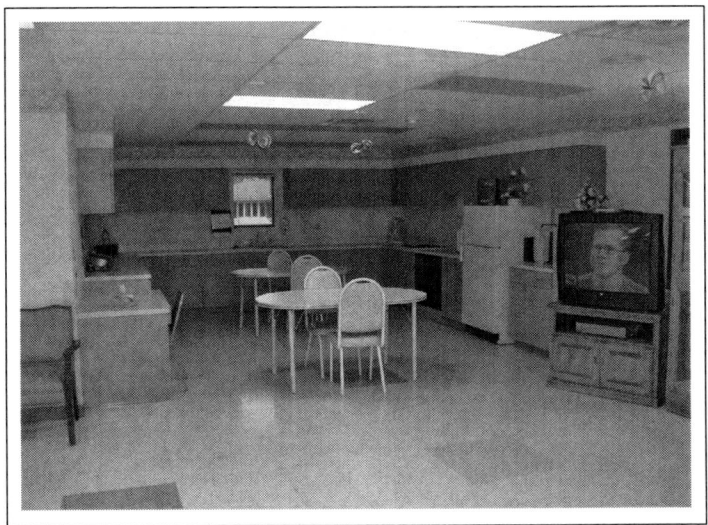

FIGURE 6.1 A Household Model

Source: Horty Elving Architectural Group.

A benchmark report for the period ending March 31, 2011, revealed that 286 of 319 facilities (89.7%) had not begun to address the development of households within their long-term care settings (Pioneer Network, 2011).

Private Rooms

> Benchmark: Percentage of residents in private rooms.

The concept of shared rooms has traditionally been an economic decision made by operators of long-term care facilities. Studies have identified, however, a direct correlation between homes with a high quality of life and homes with the most private rooms (Kane, 2004). In addition, research has found evidence to suggest that the benefits of private rooms include a number of clinical outcomes, such as lower infection rates, improved psychosocial outcomes (preferences for privacy and quality time for family visits, especially during one's end of life), and more personal control over one's space (Calkins & Casella, 2007; Cutler & Kane, 2004, 2009; Kaplan, 1983). Benefits also include a number of organizational factors, such as less time spent managing roommate conflicts. Private rooms are also easier to market to prospective residents. Several models of household and smaller living units have proven to be cost effective over time because people report higher levels of satisfaction with the facility and there is less turnover and fewer lost bed-stay days when private rooms are available (Calkins & Casella, 2007). A benchmark report for the period ending March 31, 2011, revealed that 286 of 319 facilities (89.7%) had only partially begun to address the development of private rooms for residents (Pioneer Network, 2011). Figure 6.2 provides an illustration of a home where one of the walls was knocked out to create more space and a private room. The "before" photo (6.2A) includes two residents sharing the same room, and the "after" photo (6.2B) shows how the new, larger room provides more space and privacy for one person.

Privacy-Enhanced Rooms

> Benchmark: Percentage of residents in privacy-enhanced shared rooms where residents can access their own space without trespassing through the other resident's space. This does not include the traditional privacy curtain.

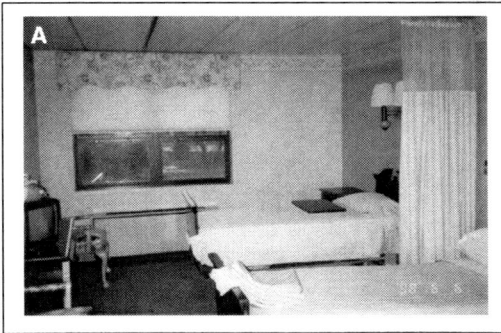

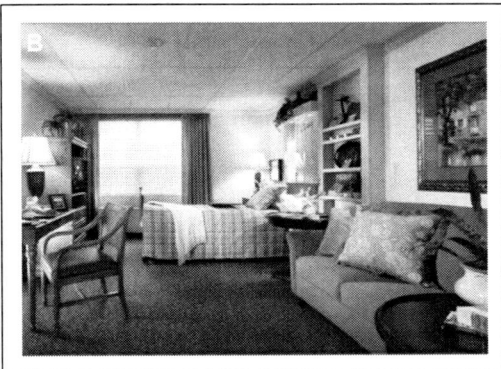

FIGURE 6.2 Images of a Private Room. (A) Before; (B) After

Source: Quality Therapy & Consultation, Inc.

A privacy-enhanced shared room has a separate living space and quarter for each individual that can be separated by a privacy wall (rather than a curtain); however, the unit can have one shared bathroom. In addition, each resident can have his or her own window and separate closet. Ideally within these types of situations, residents do not need to travel across each other's space.

Studies have revealed that residents like these enhanced rooms because it gives them a feeling that they have privacy but yet someone is still available to them. Within these types of settings, staff also report that there are fewer instances of roommate conflict (Haider, 2001; Kane et al., 2005; SAFERFoundation, 2012).

Figure 6.3 provides an illustration of this type of room setup. The privacy divider is actually a television wall unit, which provides privacy between two residents but also provides the opportunity for some shared space between them.

A benchmark report for the period ending March 31, 2011, revealed that 228 of 319 facilities (71.5%) had not begun to address this approach to creating privacy between residents who shared space with each other (Pioneer Network, 2011).

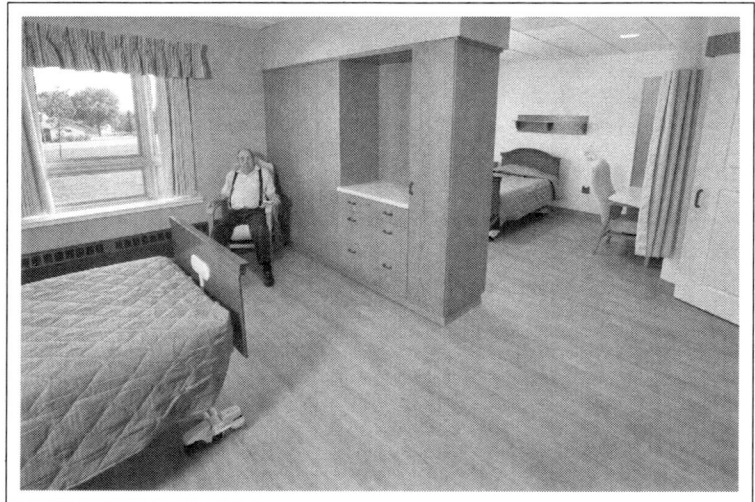

FIGURE 6.3 Residence Double Room With Privacy Divider
Source: Horty Elving Architectural Group.

Traditional Nurses' Stations

Benchmark: No traditional nurses's stations exist, or the traditional nurses' stations have been removed and transformed into some alternate space.

Although this benchmark refers to the fact that traditional nurses' stations have not been removed, the ideal is to renovate these stations so that they do not convey a separation between the resident and staff. Dispensing with the nurses' station moves the facility away from an institutional look and toward a neighborhood or household setting. This has been an area that many facilities have tackled. Kane and colleagues (2004) found that the nurses' stations were identified as an environmental problem area and recommended that the high counters be removed because they appear to separate the residents and staff.

Some potential solutions to this benchmark include disbanding the nurses' station altogether and simply using the tables in the dining room, and then leaving resident charts in a locked cabinet. Figures 6.4 and 6.5 provide illustrations of efforts to dispense with the nurses' station. Some facilities that have successfully dispensed with the nurses' station include the Village, in Indianola, IA; the Special Care Center at Health Hill, located in Oshkosh, WI; and the Green Houses, in Tupelo, MS (Schoeneman & Bowman, 2006).

Figure 6.4 illustrates what a typical nurse's station space might look like, encompassing a large amount of space, whereas Figure 6.5 portrays

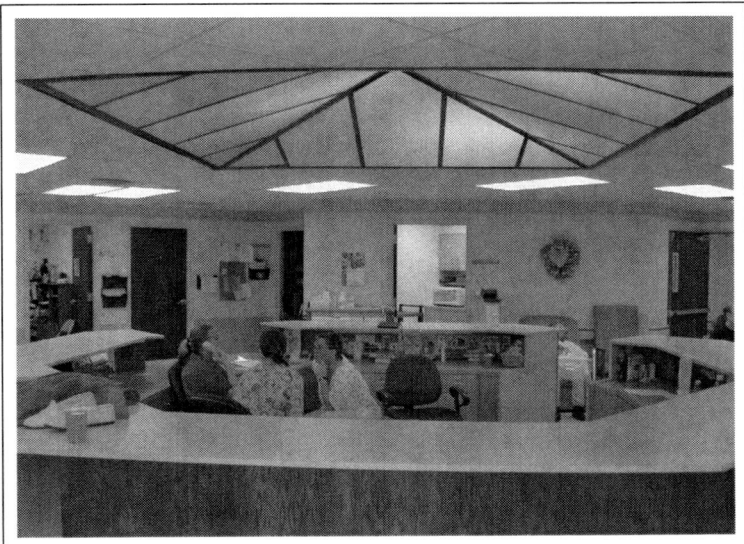

FIGURE 6.4 Traditional Nurses' Station

Source: Horty Elving Architectural Group.

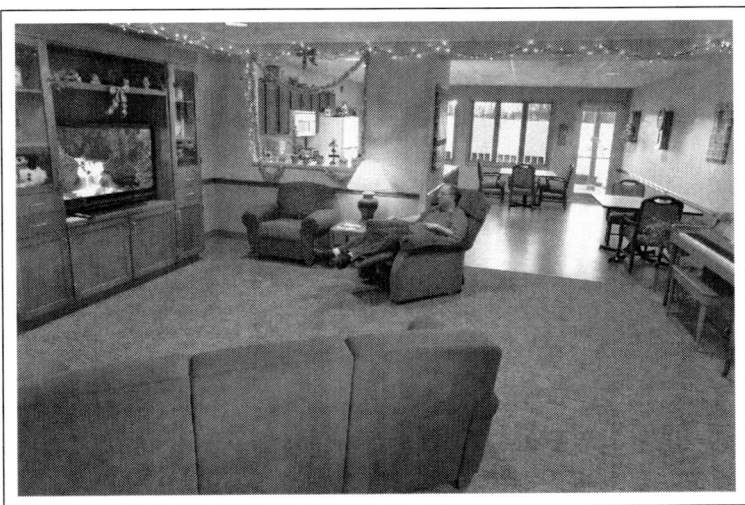

FIGURE 6.5 Nurses' Station Reworked to Provide Renovated Dining. The Dining Area Provides a Workplace for the Nurses and Has Replaced the Traditional Nurses' Station

Source: Horty Elving Architectural Group.

what this kind of space could look like after being renovated. The nurses' station now consists of a small charting area, as can be found in the left-hand side of the photo. In this setting, the nurses are found in the open with residents and, because of the space, are much more inclined to interact with residents.

Windows

> Benchmark: Percent of residents who have a direct window view not past another resident's bed.

The benchmark for windows in facilities is regarded as the percentage of residents who have a direct window view not past another resident's bed. Nursing homes commonly have a room that consists of two beds, with one bed accessing one window, and the other bed may not have access to the window if a privacy curtain is pulled shut. This could often cause conflict between roommates, especially if one wants privacy while the other wants a view. Research has identified positive outcomes for surgical patients with a hospital room view (Ulrich, 2006), including shorter bed stays, lower costs, fewer medications, better emotional well-being, and fewer minor complications (Brawley, 1997, 2006). It would be ideal if rooms had approximately the same square footage, with a window available to each bed.

A benchmark report for the period ending March 31, 2011, revealed that 174 of 319 facilities (54.5%) had partially begun to address the need for individual windows in rooms (Pioneer Network, 2011).

Bathroom Mirrors

> Benchmark: Resident bathroom mirrors are wheelchair accessible and/or adjustable in order to be visible to a seated or standing resident.

This benchmark calls attention to the position of mirrors, especially for residents in wheelchairs. Ideally, the residents' bathroom mirrors should be wheelchair accessible and/or adjustable in order to be visible to a seated or standing resident. If the mirror is not wheelchair accessible, residents may not be able to see their entire face or upper body. Although this is an easy fix, a quality of life study of nearly 2,000 residents living in 40 homes revealed that only 10% had a mirror suitable for a wheelchair user (Cutler, Kane, Degenholtz, Miller, & Grant, 2006). Figure 6.6 provides an image of a wheelchair-accessible mirror and a nonaccessible mirror.

The bathroom mirror is an example of an item that can be purchased at a local hardware store as opposed to a hospital supply company.

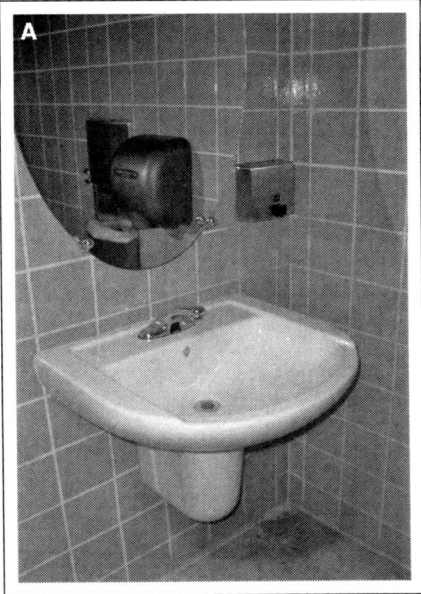 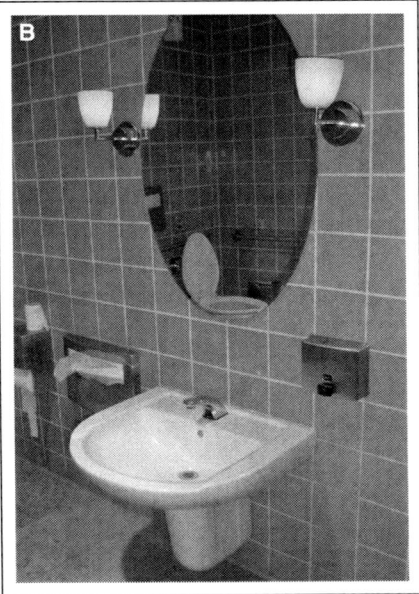

FIGURE 6.6 Bathroom Mirrors. Wheelchair-Accessible (A); Nonaccessible due to the height of the mirror (B)

Source: Tuscany Village Nursing and Rehabilitation Center.

Facilities that do not have a union shop responsible for the physical plan can easily look for volunteers from their team or family members to help with the renovation of bathroom fixtures. These contributions of labor can be of much help to the overall facility budget and operating expenses.

A benchmark report for the period ending March 3, 2011, revealed that 187 of 319 facilities (58.6%) had addressed this in full (Pioneer Network, 2011).

Wheelchair-Accessible Sinks

Benchmark: Sinks in resident bathrooms are wheelchair accessible, with clearance below sinks for wheelchairs.

Another area of concern in the bathroom includes accessible sinks. This benchmark calls for sinks in resident bathrooms to be wheelchair accessible, with clearance below the sink for a wheelchair. Although I recommend that facilities have wheelchair-accessible equipment, it is also a very important idea to check the local city code for the specifications required for the sink to be wheelchair accessible and for washstands to meet the standards mandated by the Architectural Barriers Act and the Americans with Disabilities Act.

Cutler et al. (2006) found that 82% of long-term care facilities had adequate wheelchair clearance under their sinks. A benchmark report for the period ending March 31, 2011, revealed that 268 of 319 facilities (84%) had met this goal (Pioneer Network, 2011).

Adaptive Sinks

> Benchmark: Sinks used by residents have adaptive/easy-to-use lever or paddle handles.

This benchmark calls for sinks used by residents to have adaptive/easy-to-use lever or paddle handles, which is a relatively quick fix. Most facilities rarely have lever-style paddle handles installed, but this adaptation is easy to see to completion. Most hardware stores have easy access to paddle and lever hardware these days. Cutler and Kane (2004) suggested that hardware stores such as Home Depot or Lowes can probably provide more economical options to help adapt sinks rather than securing the equipment from a long-term care supplier. A benchmark report for the period ending March 3, 2011, revealed that 207 of 319 facilities (64.9%) had fully met this goal (Pioneer Network, 2011). Figure 6.7 provides an illustration of a wheelchair-accessible sink, and Figure 6.8 provides illustrations of examples of adaptive sinks.

Adaptive Door Handles

> Benchmark: Adaptive handles, enhanced for easy use, are positioned on doors used by residents (e.g., in resident rooms, bathrooms, and public areas).

Adaptive handles, enhanced for easy use, for doors used by residents (e.g. in their rooms, bathrooms, and public areas) is another benchmark that can remedy an environment for people with limited physical grip. Although the numbers may have changed in recent years, only about half of the homes currently have this lever-type hardware available (Cutler & Kane, 2004). These lever devices can also be found in a

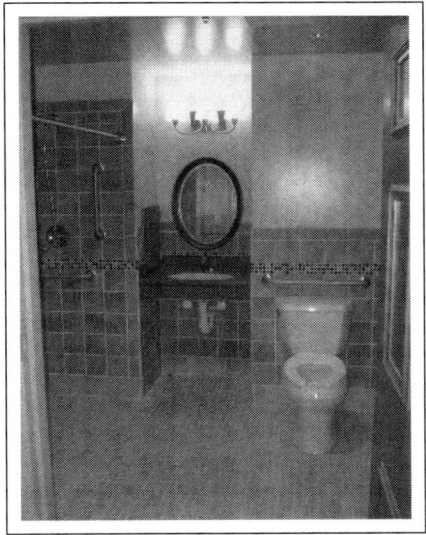

FIGURE 6.7 Wheelchair-Accessible Sink

Source: Tuscany Village Long Term Care Center.

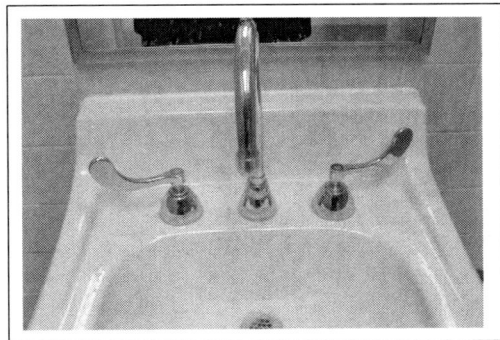 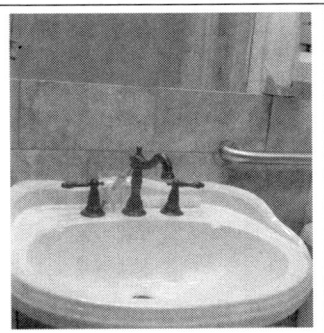

FIGURE 6.8 Adaptive Sinks

cost-effective manner through local hardware stores, as opposed to a more costly institutional supply company.

Closets

Benchmark: Closets have movable rods that can be set to different heights.

Ideally, closets should have movable rods that can be set to different heights, so people, regardless of height or wheelchair use, can access their clothing in the closet. In 2004, Kane found that only 6.9% of facilities surveyed met this benchmark. Cutler (2006) found that only 7% of facility residents surveyed were able to access clothing in their closets because of the position of the closet rods. A benchmark report for the period ending March 31, 2011, revealed that 260 of 319 (81.5%) of facilities had met this goal in full (Pioneer Network, 2011). Thus, progress is on the horizon!

Room Décor

> Benchmark: The facility has no rule prohibiting room décor and residents are welcome to decorate their rooms any way they wish, including using nails, tape, screws, and so on.

Room décor helps create a personal space that helps identify who a person is and what is unique about his or her personality. It helps establish identity and individuality. Room décor includes the color of the room, trim used around the room, pictures, furnishings, and lighting. This benchmark prescribes that homes have no rule that prohibits residents from personalizing the décor of their surroundings. Residents are welcome to decorate their rooms any way they wish, including using nails, tape, screws, and other materials. Figure 6.9 is an example of an altimeter clock from a room where the resident was a former pilot.

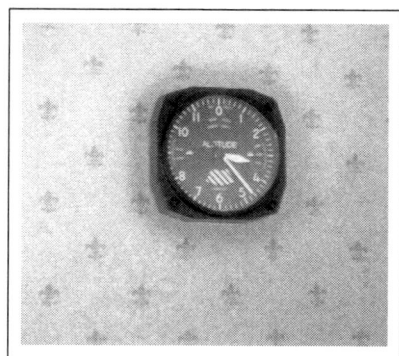

FIGURE 6.9 An Example of Personalizing a Resident's Room

Source: Tuscany Village Nursing Center.

Ideally, people should be allowed to decorate with their own furnishings, their own photos, and so on, down to the bed sheets and linens. All too often, rooms have the traditional white or beige tones. Consider color for individual rooms and wallpaper features to add life and individuality.

Cutler and Kane (2004) identified a host of innovations that can help residents create their own space and add personalized touches to their room. The entrance should be reminiscent of a house that one has always wanted to be invited into. This can include, for example, painting the door frame a different color than the wall to help cue the individual resident that it is his or her room. An individual mailbox can be installed at each door. Furnishings that create a living space instead of just a "sleeping space" can also individualize a resident's room and create a homelike culture. The use of light can help to individualize a room and create a more positive ambience. Floor lamps and desk lamps can be helpful and can be easily accessed through the use of remote controls. Bins can be used in storage spaces. A benchmark report for the period ending March 31, 2011, revealed that 260 of 319 (81.5%) of facilities had met this goal in full (Pioneer Network, 2011), which suggests that this approach may be an easier goal to meet than some of the other goals within the series of benchmarks.

Lighting

> Benchmark: The facility makes available extra lighting sources, such as floor lamps and/or reading lamps, in residents' rooms if requested by a resident.

As one grows older, the sensitivity to and need for lighting becomes increasingly important. Because the retina is not as thin in an older adult as in a younger person, lighting can play a role in helping people see clearly in their surroundings or be able to read. This benchmark calls for homes to make extra lighting sources, such as floor and/or reading lamps, available in residents' rooms if requested by a resident. Although the expectation is for the home to provide this amenity, individuals often will purchase floor lamps on their own. Lighting can take the form of fixtures, floor lamps, table lamps, and nightlights. Nightlights may be a good option for people who would like some light but do not wish to have a floor lamp on all night.

A benchmark report for the period ending March 31, 2011, revealed that 250 of 319, or 78.4%, of facilities had met this goal in full (Pioneer Network, 2011).

Heat/Air Conditioning

> Benchmark: Heat/air conditioning controls can be adjusted in residents' rooms.

This benchmark addresses personal control of one's heat/air conditioning settings. A quality of life study conducted by Cutler et al. in 2006 revealed that only 52% of residents' rooms had adjustable heat, and 46% had adjustable air conditioning. In contrast, by 2011, 195 of 319 (61.1%) facilities surveyed had met this goal in full (Pioneer Network, 2011).

Refrigerators

> Benchmark: The facility provides or invites residents to have their own refrigerators.

Personal access to a refrigerator can enable residents to have a preferred snack any time of day or night. It also allows family members to bring specialty or ethnic dishes to the facility. To meet this benchmark, the facility or home provides or invites residents to have their own refrigerators within their rooms. Bump (2005) suggested that food is intertwined with every aspect of one's being, and with access to a personal refrigerator and microwave people can feel like they have their own mini-kitchen. In Cutler's (2006) quality-of-life study of nearly 2,000 residents, only 1.5% had access to a refrigerator in facilities/homes. This stands in contrast to recent findings from the Pioneer Network in 2011 that indicated that 189 of 319 (59.2%) of facilities permitted residents to have a personal refrigerator or had a policy that allowed for these personal effects.

Chairs and Sofas

> Benchmark: Chairs and sofas in public areas have varied seat heights to comfortably accommodate people of different heights.

As people grow older, their need for seating that is firm enough to let them support themselves as they get out of a seated position becomes increasingly important. This benchmark calls for chairs and sofas in public areas to have seat heights that vary to comfortably accommodate people of different heights. A 6-foot male would need a different height of chair than a 4-foot, 9-inch woman; however, both may reside in the same home. The Americans with Disabilities Act of 1990 recommends that seating heights be between 17.5 and 18.5 inches. Unfortunately, not all older adults (or even younger adults) are about the same height, so this guideline may result in uncomfortable seating. Cushions can help accommodate height as well as chairs that are too deep. Chairs with arms that are well supported are preferable because these offer support to people as they push themselves up from a seated position. This benchmark seems more difficult to accomplish, and only 120 of 319 facilities (37.6%) reported that they had partially met this goal in the most recent survey (Pioneer Network, 2011).

Gliders

Benchmark: Gliders that lock into place when the person rises are available inside the home and/or outside.

Gliders are a form of rocking chair commonly used in homelike settings. Ideally, a glider that locks into place when the person rises should be available inside the home and/or outside for use, according to this benchmark. The locking position makes the chair more stable for easy entry and exit. Although gliders may seem like an added luxury, evidence suggests that they improve one's emotions and significantly improve one's relaxation after as little as 10 minutes in the chair (Snyder et al., 2001). Other benefits to the use of gliders include increased circulation, because the rocking motion can redistribute and recycle the pressure between the resident's seat and back. Rocking also has a stimulating effect on the vestibular canal in one's ear, which can create a calming effect (Brawley, 1997). Rockers can also provide some relief to people with Alzheimer's disease, who can be aggressive; rocking has been known to be calming and therapeutic (Brawley, 1997). Of the homes responding to a benchmark survey by the Pioneer Network in 2011, 239 of 319 (74.9%) reported no use of gliders in their homes.

Gift Shop

> Benchmark: The facility has a store/gift shop/cart available where residents can purchase snacks or gifts.

For some people with mobility limitations, the home-based gift shop may be the only option for finding a birthday card for a grandchild or a sympathy card to send to a grieving friend. The availability of such a shop may also be a lifeline to fill a craving when one wants a desired snack. This benchmark suggests that homes have a store/gift shop/cart available where residents can purchase snacks or gifts. Although not always practical due to staffing issues, it may serve as an opportunity for some of the higher functioning residents to work at the gift shop on a rotational basis.

Internet/Computer Access

> Benchmark: Residents have regular access to computers/the Internet, and adaptations are available for independent computer use, such as large keyboards or touch screens.

Increasingly, people growing older will expect access to computers and/or the Internet. In today's digital age, it is rare to find an older adult with grandchildren who do not use a computer. Currently, the oldest-old and most frail may not have had access to the computer or the Internet in their lifetimes, but baby boomers will certainly expect these resources. Outcome studies suggest that when older adults in homes have access to the computer and the Internet, they increase communications with their family, increase their socialization with other residents and staff, improve their self-esteem, increase attendance at group activities, decrease agitation, and improve self-expression (Dow et al., 2008; Dunning, 2011; Nycyk & Redsell, 2011). Teaching residents how to use a computer, connect to social networking sites, and use the Internet are excellent intergenerational opportunities. Volunteers from local high schools, community colleges, or universities can be an excellent resource to meet this need in homes. In addition, Skype provides a wonderful way for older adults to connect with their loved ones, such as children, grandchildren, and great-grandchildren. Helping residents with communication on the Internet can be wonderful service projects for local Girl Scout or Boy Scout troops.

The Pioneer Network benchmark survey (2011) revealed that, of the 319 facilities that reported results, 126 (39.4%) had partially met this goal.

Workout Room

> Benchmark: A workout room is available to residents.

Access to movement and varying forms of exercise are important for people at any age, but particularly for older adults who already are limited in their mobility. To help meet fitness and mobility goals, a benchmark to have a workout room available to residents was established. Although older adults may be fearful of using equipment, there are strategies to introduce the equipment and the concept of working out in a manner that is not strenuous. Exercise has been proven to have multiple benefits for older adults. Symptoms of depression, functional performance, and muscle strength were all positively impacted through a progressive functional fitness/strength training program (Brill et al., 2011). Kuiak et al. (2003) found that a structured resistive training program that was implemented with older people who had dementia improved muscle strength and power.

Figure 6.10 provides an overview of workout rooms in facilities located in Minnesota (Rice Care, located in Willmar, MN and MN Veteran's Home located in Warroad, MN). These rooms have been so popular that people line up to use the machines. One of the residents, frustrated with the wait, donated a piece of workout equipment to help ease the lineup.

Bathing Rooms

> Benchmark: Bathing rooms have functional and properly installed heat lamps, radiant heat panels, or the equivalent.

Bathing areas can be perceived as uncomfortable because of the sudden temperature changes between the air and the bathwater. This rapid temperature difference can leave people somewhat resistant to taking showers or baths. The Artifacts for Culture Change Tool benchmark for bathing calls for rooms that have functional and properly installed heat

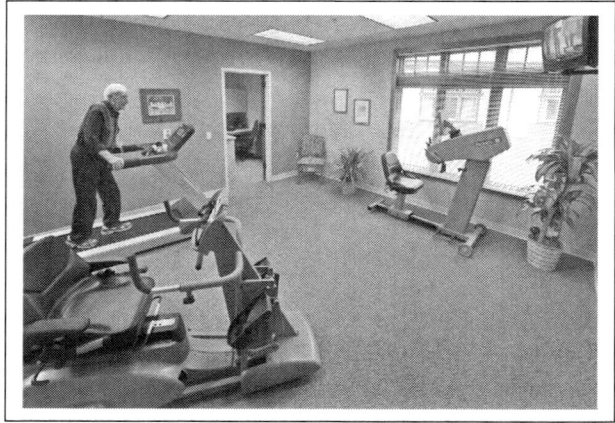

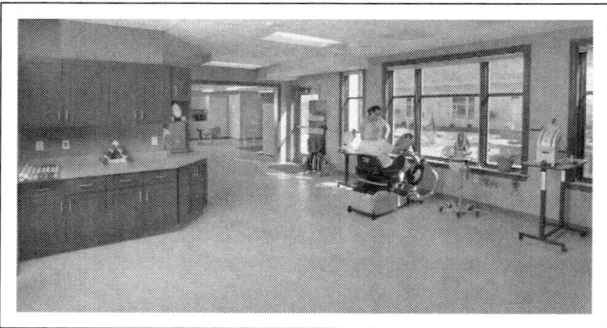

FIGURE 6.10 Workout Rooms

Source: Horty Elving Architectural Group.

lamps and radiant heat panels or the equivalent. Heat lamps can be easily installed, along with bathtubs that do not appear to be institutional. Figure 6.11 provides some illustrations to address this point.

An innovative way to shift from the bathing experience to something more positive could be to rename the bathing experience the "spa experience" or "spa time." The actual signage could read "Spa Room." Bowman (2005) recommended that items stored in the room that do not enhance the bathing experience should be removed from the room. If need be, clean and repaint the room, and re-grout or shine the tiled surfaces. Sink faucets can be replaced with single-lever handles. Stencils or other wall painting can be used to enhance the ambience of the room. Storage units can also enhance the room and can be purchased at a low cost from local hardware goods stores. Items such as a wall shelf, glass door cabinets, or rolling carts can be used to store towels. Towel colors can also be coordinated with the tile and decorations to move away from an institutional approach to one that is homelike.

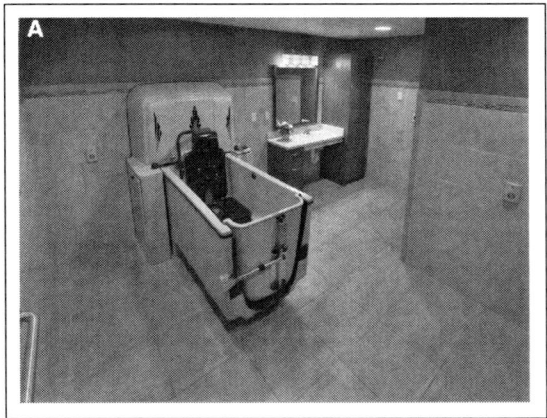

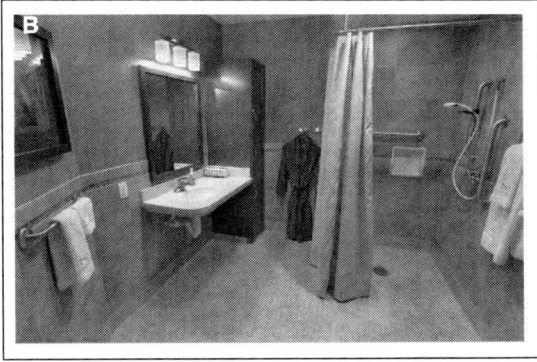

FIGURE 6.11 (A) Therapy Suites, Rice Care Spa. (B) Therapy Suites, Rice Care Resident's Bath.

Source: Horty Elving Architectural Group

Towels

Benchmark: The facility warms towels for resident bathing.

Warmed bath towels can enhance the bathing experience. Another benchmark related to bathing suggests that the home warms towels for resident bathing. This is not an expensive fix and can be accomplished with towel warmers for under $500. Facilities may want to follow the example set by the Fort Collins Good Samaritan Home, in Fort Collins, CO, which provides warm towels to residents at all times with their mid-sized industrial towel warmer. Despite the fact that this is a relatively simple fix, the Pioneer Network benchmark survey (2011) revealed that, of the 319 facilities that reported results, 225 (70.5%) had not met this goal at all.

Outdoor Garden/Patio

> Benchmark: A protected outdoor garden/patio is accessible for independent use by residents.

Residents, including those who use wheelchairs, should be able to enter and exit the facility independently; that is, they should not need assistance from staff to open doors or overcome obstacles in traveling to the patio.

Many older adults living in long-term care facilities have had the opportunity in the past to own homes and maintain outdoor gardens and patios. Consequently, this benchmark encourages care facilities to have a protected outdoor garden/patio accessible for independent use by residents. Cultivating an outdoor space for residents helps them connect to their environment and to nature. It also increases the likelihood that they will socialize with others and stay involved in outdoor activities. Cutler and Kane (2006) found that several hours of outdoor activity in the morning had a tremendous impact on reducing unwanted behaviors later in the day. Outdoor spaces are as critical as indoor spaces, and planning to ensure their functionality and accessibility, especially for wheelchairs, walkers, and other mobility devices, is important.

Bird feeders, sun umbrellas, and so on can provide a less sterile approach to either enclosed porches or sitting room areas. Adequate protection from the sun is also essential in facilitating the use of the porch area.

Figure 6.12 provides an after picture of an outdoor space and illustrates how the space had been renovated at a facility in northern Minnesota. Urban legend tales shared by residents and staff quickly explained the orange cones lined up alongside the garden porch area. According to the stories, a resident with her walker had been hit by a car backing up the driveway (M. Jeaneau, personal communication, June 16, 2012). Thus, the cones were placed to protect people from moving beyond the safe zone. Culture change efforts in this facility led to a screened-in porch that is usable for at least three seasons of the year and

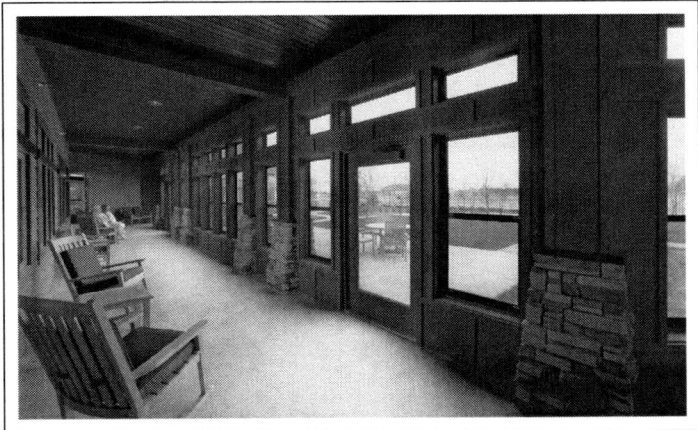

FIGURE 6.12 Front Porch, Enclosed to Accommodate Use for Three Seasons

Source: Horty Elving Architectural Group.

that provides a dimension of privacy and protection from the elements for residents and their family members.

Outdoor Raised Gardens

> Benchmark: The facility has outdoor, raised gardens available for resident use.

In addition to the outdoor garden/patio benchmark, an additional benchmark recommends that homes have outdoor, raised gardens available for resident use. Raised gardens (garden beds that are set 3–4 feet above the ground) can give older adults and residents a renewed sense of success, improve their self-confidence, and promote self-esteem (Kwatch et al., 2004). Well-designed raised gardens can help people maintain their green thumb, despite their mobility and access limitations (Kwatch et al., 2004). Kane et al. (2004) found this benchmark to be a problem area, because 32% of the residents they surveyed went outdoors less than once a month, 13% went less than once a week. Although the concept of outdoor activities involving gardening and raised planters is a good one, residents often had difficulty navigating themselves in their wheelchairs on the outdoor surfaces. A consideration to be made with the gardens is to ensure that nontoxic plants are used, especially so that people with dementia are not affected by their tasting habits!

Figure 6.13 provides an illustration of a patio converted area.

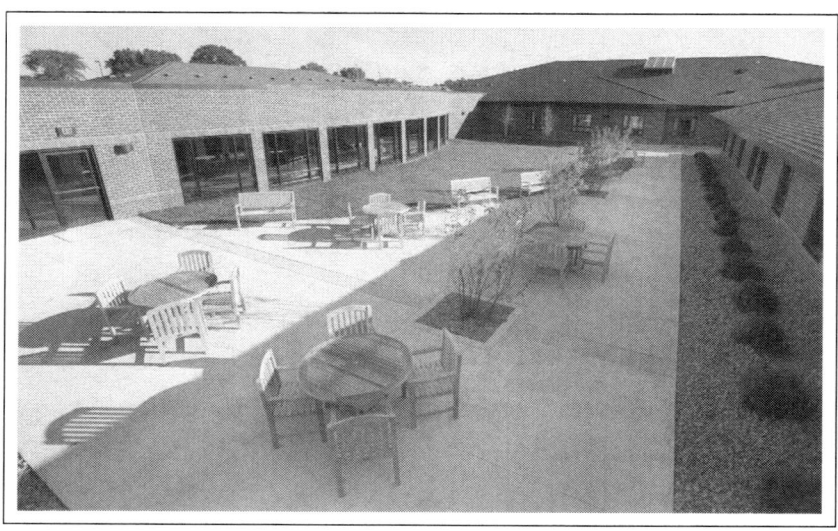

FIGURE 6.13 Garden/Patio Setting
Source: Horty Elving Architectural Group.

Outdoor Walking/Wheeling Path

> Benchmark: The facility has an outdoor walking/wheeling path that is not a city sidewalk or path.

This benchmark suggests that homes have an outdoor walking/wheeling path that is not a city sidewalk or path. A benchmark report for the period ending March 31, 2011, revealed that 251 of 319 facilities (78.6%) had partially met this goal (Pioneer Network, 2011).

Pager/Radio/Call System

> Benchmark: A pager/radio/telephone call system is used whereby resident calls register on staffs' pagers/radios/telephones and staff can use them to communicate with fellow staff.

A pager/radio/telephone call system is used whereby resident calls register on staffs' pagers/radios/telephones and staff can use them to communicate with fellow staff. Eliminating distracting announcements through the facility is the goal that this benchmark addresses. The concept of a wireless call system seems to be gaining ground within the culture change movement and appears to be a tool to be used to promote better services and a more calming effect. Residents can find comfort in an environment that is devoid of ringing and the flashing of call lights (Bowman, 2005).

Emergency Paging

> Benchmark: The facility's overhead paging system has been turned off or is only used in case of emergency.

One of the major benefits of this approach is that facilities have a greatly reduced level of white noise throughout the building. This reduction in noise mitigates resident agitation, improves the working environment, increases resident privacy, and creates a more normalized living environment for all (Brokaw, 2006).

Laundry

> Benchmark: Personal clothing is laundered on resident household/neighborhood/ units instead of in a general all-home laundry, and residents/families have access to a washer and dryer for their own use.

Within the realm of laundry, the benchmark or goal is that personal clothing is laundered on resident household/neighborhood/units instead of in a general all-home laundry, and residents/families have access to a washer and dryer for their own use. This approach has two main positive outcomes. First, laundry done on a smaller residential unit leaves fewer opportunities to lose clothes, because staff can more likely identify a resident's item. Second, laundering within the unit also helps to reduce unnecessarily wrinkling, because the clothing will likely not be transported any great distance.

OTHER FEATURES

Two additional areas that provide an overall look and feel of a homelike environment are the hallways and entranceways. Hallways have traditionally been cluttered with equipment, wheelchairs, or other unsightly materials. Options are available to distract from the "institutional appeal" and create a more homelike setting. Closets or storage spaces can be created along corridors to conceal wheelchairs or Hoyer lifts. Figure 6.14 provides "before" images of a home, with equipment cluttering the hallway, and Figure 6.15 provides illustrations of renovated space, with closet spaces along the corridor for adaptive equipment.

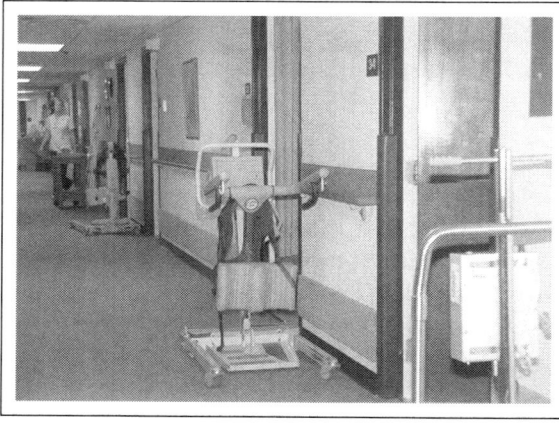

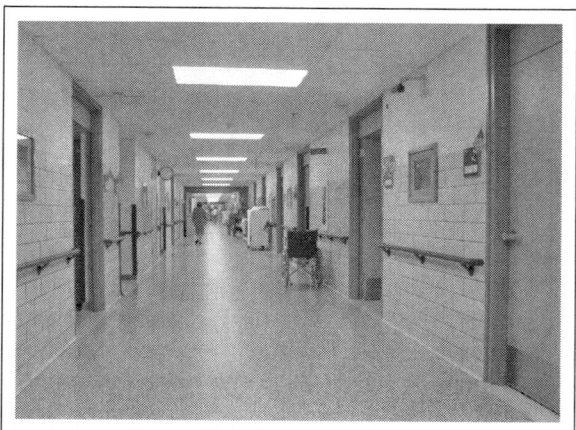

FIGURE 6.14   Hallway Photos Prior to Renovation

Source: Horty Elving Architectural Group.

A second area of note is probably the most critical, because it sets the tone for facilities—the entryway. Ideally, this area should be welcoming, and provide a sense that one is entering a space filled with comfort and life, rather than being dilapidated looking. Some examples of these types of environments and entrances are illustrated in Figures 6.16 and 6.17.

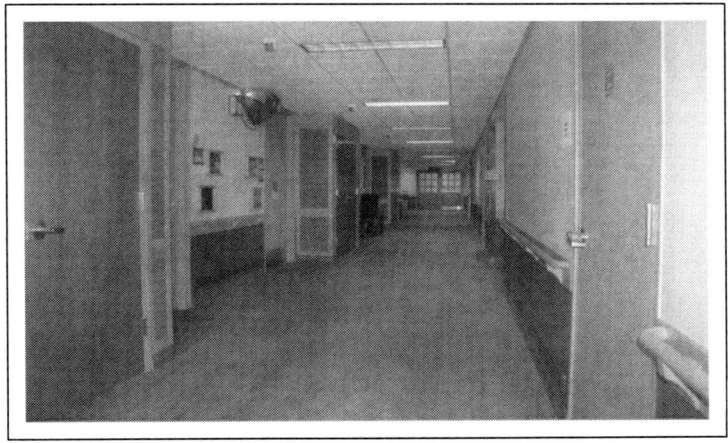

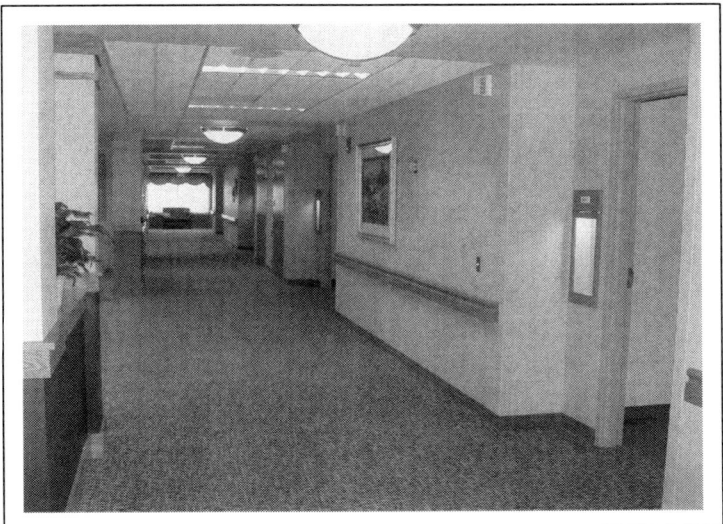

FIGURE 6.15 Hallway Photos (Same Angle as Figure 6.14) After Renovation

Source: Horty Elving Architectural Group.

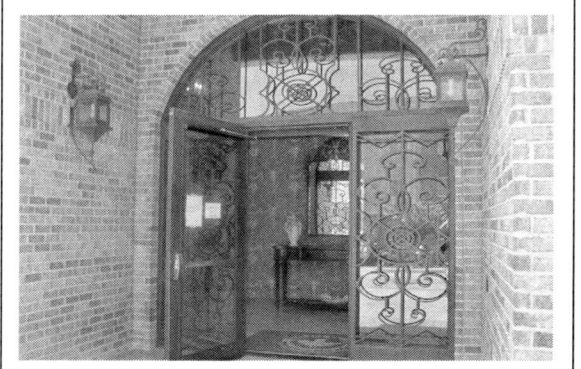
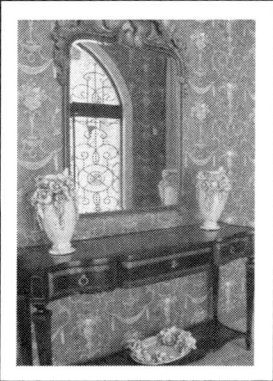
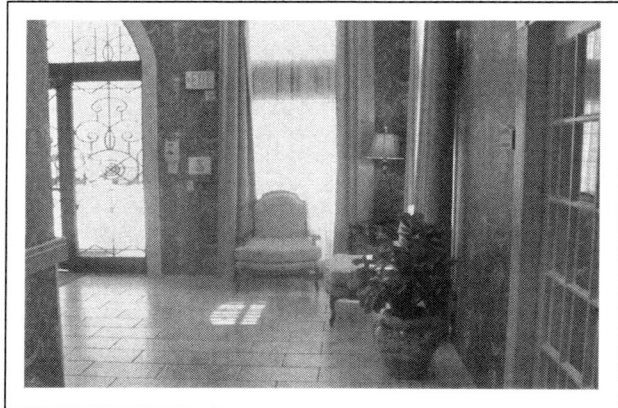
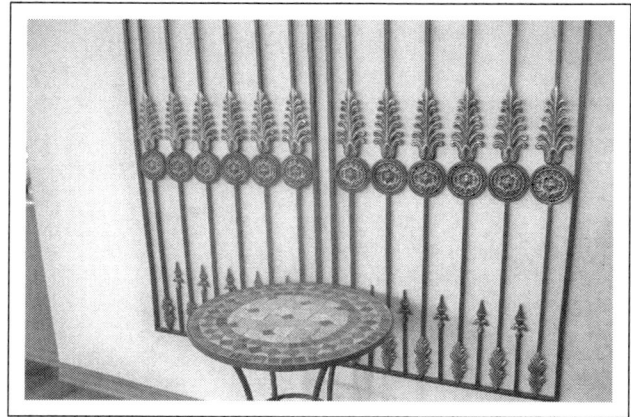

FIGURE 6.16 Examples of Entrances

Source: Tuscany Village and Rehabilitation Center.

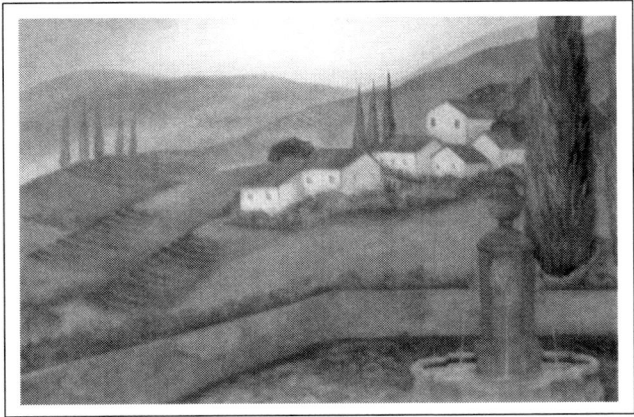

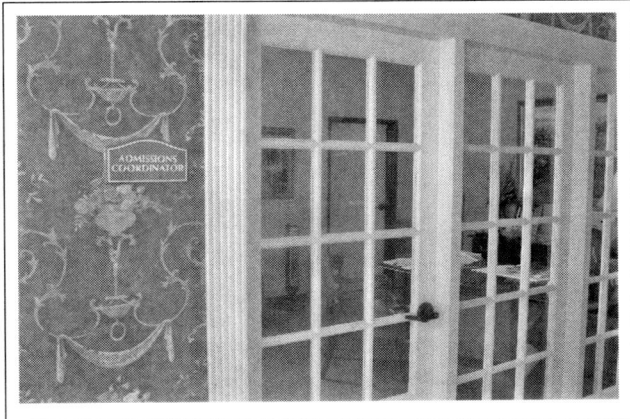

FIGURE 6.17 Mural and Entry Areas

Source: Tuscany Village and Rehabilitation Center.

SUMMARY

This chapter addressed strategies and benchmarks to enhance the environment and create a homelike approach to long-term care settings. At the outset of the chapter, I reviewed the importance of environment on one's functioning and adaptation. Throughout the chapter, benchmarks to be met in an effort to implement a culture change paradigm within long-term care settings were reviewed, and strategies to address these benchmarks were presented.

DISCUSSION/REFLECTION QUESTIONS

1. Identify five specific benchmark items presented in this chapter that you would not have thought of prior to reading the chapter. How do these environmental benchmarks shape the environment to be more in line with a culture change paradigm?
2. Identify five benchmarks within the environment domain that you feel have been met within facilities in which you either worked or to which you have been exposed. Explain why you feel these benchmarks were met.
3. Identify three strategies that you and your team could use to address at least one (or up to three) specific benchmarks in the environment domain.
4. Think about a service learning project in which you and your classmates or colleagues could get involved to help a local facility (or the facility in which you currently work) to help meet one of the benchmarks in the environment domain. What steps will you need to put into place to accomplish this goal?

REFERENCES

Baumeister, R. F., & Tice, D. M. (1985). Self-esteem and responses to success and failure: Subsequent performance and intrinsic motivation. *Journal of Personality 53*, 450–67.

Bowman, C. (2005). Wireless gains ground. *Culture Change Now, 3*, 13.

Bowman, C. (2008, April). *The environmental side of the culture change movement: Identifying barriers and potential solutions to furthering innovation in nursing homes.* Pre-symposium background paper presented at "Creating Home in the Nursing Home: A National Symposium on Culture Change and the Environment Requirements," Washington, DC.

Brawley, E. (1997). *Designing for Alzheimer's disease: Strategies for creating better care environments.* New York, NY: Wiley.

Brawley, E. C. (2006). *Design innovations for aging and Alzheimer's.* John Wiley & Sons, Inc.

Brill, P., Jensen, R., Koltyn, K., Morgan, L., Morrow, J., Keller, M., & Jackson, A. (2011). The feasibility of conducting a group-based progressive strength training program in residents of a multi-level care facility. *Activities, Adaptations and Aging, 22*, 53–63.

Brokaw, G. (2006). CEO Fairport Baptist Home, correspondence dated 4/3/2006. Fairport, NY.

Bump, L. (2005). The process of physical design: Regulations and the physical design. *Culture Change Now, 3*, 10–17.

Calkins, M., & Casella, C. (2007). Exploring the cost and value of private versus shared bedrooms in nursing homes. *The Gerontologist, 47*, 169–183.

Calkins, M., Kator, M., Wyatt, A., & Halliday, L. (2009). Culture change in action: Changing the experiential environment. *Long Term Living: For the Continuing Care Professional, 58*, 16.

Cutler, L. J. (2000). Assessing the environment of older adults. In R. L. Kane & R. A. Kane (Eds.), *Assessing older adults* (pp. 360–379). Oxford, UK: Oxford University Press.

Cutler, L. J. (2006). Assessing and comparing physical environments for nursing home residents: Using new tool for greater specificity. *The Gerontologist, 46*(1). 42–51.

Cutler, L. J. (2007). Physical environments of assisted living: Research needs and challenges. *The Gerontologist, 47*(suppl 1), 68–82.

Cutler, L. J., & Kane, R. A (2004). *Practical strategies to transform nursing home environments: Towards a better quality of life manual*. Minneapolis, MN: University of Minnesota Press.

Cutler, L. J., & Kane, R. A. (2006). As great as all outdoors: A study of outdoor spaces as a neglected resource for nursing home residents. *Journal of Housing for the Elderly, 9*, 3–4.

Cutler, L. J., & Kane, R. A. (2009). Post occupancy evaluation of a transformed nursing home: The first four Green House settings. *Journal of Housing for the Elderly, 23*, 304–334.

Cutler, L. J., Kane, R. A., Degenholtz, H. B., Miller, M. J., & Grant, L. (2006). Assessing and comparing the physical environments for nursing home residents: Using new tools for greater research specificity. *The Gerontologist, 46*, 42–51.

Dow, B., Moore, K., Scott, P., Ratnayeke, A., Wise, J., Simms, J., & Hill, K. (2008). Rural carers online: A feasibility study. *Australian Journal of Rural Health, 16*, 221–225. doi:10.1111/j.1440-1584.2008.00982:x

Dunning, T. A. (2011). *A resident computer lab: Participation and outcomes. Christian Living Campus*, Denver, CO. Unpublished manuscript.

Haider, E. (2001). Crestview Manor, Bethany, MO.

Howard, D., Nieuwenhuijsen, E. R., & Saleeby, P. (2008). Health promotion and education: Application of the *ICF* in the US and Canada using an ecological perspective. *Disability and Rehabilitation, 30*, 942–954. doi:10.1080/09638280701800483

Kahana, E. (1975). A congruence model of person environment interaction. In P. G. Windley, T. Byherts, & E. G. Ernst (Eds.), *Theoretical development in environments and aging*. Washington, DC: Gerontological Society.

Kane, R. (2004). *Measures, indicators and improvement of quality of life in nursing homes: Final report*. Baltimore, MD: Centers for Medicare & Medicaid Services.

Kane, R. A. (2003). Definition, measurement, and correlates of quality of life in nursing homes: Towards a reasonable practice, research, and policy agenda. *The Gerontologist, 43*, 28–36.

Kane, R. L., Rockwood, T., Hyer, K., Desjardins, K., Brassard, A., Gessert, C., & Kane, R. (2005). Rating the importance of nursing home residents' quality of life. *Journal of the American Geriatrics Society, 53*(12), 2076–2082.

Kaplan, R. (1984). Impact of urban nature: A theoretical analysis. *Urban Ecology, 8*(3), 189–197.

Karls, J. M., & Wandrei, K. E. (1992). PIE: A new language for social work. *Social Work, 37*(1), 80–85.

Kuiak, S., Campbell, W., Evans, W. A. (2003). Structured resistive training program improves muscle strength and power in elderly persons with dementia. *Activities, Adaptations and Aging Journal, 28*(1), 35–47.

Kwach, H., Relf, P., Rudolph, J. (2004). Adapting garden activities for overcoming difficulties of individuals with dementia and activity limitations. *Activities, Adaptations and Aging Journal, 29*(1), 1–13.

Langer, E., & Rodin, J. (1976). The effect of choice and enhanced personal responsibility for the aged: A field experiment in an institutional setting. *Journal of Personality and Social Psychology, 34*(2), 191–198.

Lawton, M. P. (1990). Residential environment and self-directedness among older people. *American Psychologist, 45*, 638–640.

Lawton, M., Fulcomer, M., & Kleban, M. H. (1984). Architecture for the mentally impaired elderly. *Environment and Behavior, 16*, 730–757. doi:10.1177/0013916584166004

Lawton, M., & Nahemow, L. (1973). Ecology and the aging process. In C. Eisdorfer & M. Lawton (Eds.), *The psychology of adult development and aging* (pp. 619–674). Washington, DC: American Psychological Association. doi:10.1037/10044-020

Maier, S. F., & Seligman, M. E. (1976). Learned helplessness: Theory and evidence. *Journal of Experimental Psychology: General, 105*(1), 3–46.

Nycyk, M., & Redsell, M. (2011). Intergenerational relationships and community computer training: Overcoming the digital divide. *Journal of Intergenerational Relationships, 9*, 85–89.

Pioneer Network. (2011). Artifacts of Culture Change benchmark reports, 04/01/2010–03/31/2011. *Tools for Change, 1*(1).

Robinson, S. B., & Rosher, R. B. (2006). Tangling with the barriers of culture change: Creating a resident-centered nursing home environment. *Journal of Gerontological Nursing, 32*(10), 19–25.

SAFERFoundation (2012). Statistics. Retrieved May 28, 2012 from www.SAFERFoundation.org

Saleeby, P. (2007). Applications of a capability approach to disability and the *International Classification of Functioning, Disability and Health* (ICF) in social work practice. *Journal of Social Work in Disability & Rehabilitation, 60*, 217–232.

Schoeneman, K., & Bowman, C. (2006). *Development of the Artifacts of Culture Change Tool: Report of Contract HHSM-500-2005-00076P* (Technical report). Baltimore, MD: Centers for Medicaid & Medicare Services. Retrieved from http://www.artifactsofculturechange.org/Data/Documents/artifacts.pdf

Snyder, M., Tseng, Y. H., Brandt, C., Croghan, C., Hanson, S., Constantine, R., & Kirby, L. (2001). A glider swing intervention for people with dementia. *Geriatric Nursing, 22*(2), 86–90.

Ulrich, W. (2006). Critical pragmatism: A new approach to professional and business ethics. *Interdisciplinary yearbook of business ethics, 1*(13), 53–86.

7

Family and Community Practices

Family and community practices form the basis of relationships and promote a sense of community within the realm of how long-term care facilities deliver support to elderly people and people with disabilities. These practices form the basis on which many residents and their families define quality or satisfaction. In this chapter, the family and community practices identified as benchmarks in the Artifacts of Culture Change Tool (ACCT; Schoeneman & Bowman, 2006) are examined and discussed to provide ideas how some of them can be executed within the culture change paradigm. Examples from successful facilities are discussed, and strategies to help meet these specific benchmarks are identified.

THE IMPORTANCE OF FAMILY AND COMMUNITY ENGAGEMENT

Community engagement can be defined in a number of ways by the individual. It can refer to the place where one's home or residence is located, or it can refer to the sense of belonging one feels within a context or situation; it also can mean a cooperative spirit. In the long run, a sense of community will help battle loneliness and isolation; build meaningful experiences; and create a sense of meaning, belonging, and purpose (Illinois Pioneer Coalition, 2010).

Several examples of how community is conceptualized and operationalized have been developed by a host of long-term care facilities in Illinois through a recent publication entitled *Tales From the Prairie: Culture Change Practices in Illinois Long Term Care Communities* (Illinois Pioneer Coalition, 2010). Administrators at the Sheltering Oak facility, located in Island Lake, IL, decided to define community in a way specific to the facility/home. The process began at a resident council meeting where people were asked to give their definition of the word *community*. Residents and staff were all expected to participate in defining community and, over time, the word helped shape the facility's culture. Residents began talking to one another, both within and outside of meetings, and stopped talking about each other in destructive and derogatory ways (Cheng, Li, Leung, & Chan, 2011). The exercise helped the group to move away from identifying themselves as a member of a "nursing facility" to a member of a "community" (Andonian & MacRae, 2011). Thus, the power of words can begin to transform the culture of community, and has done so for at least one facility.

Fostering relationships is an important dynamic in creating a culture of community. This can begin through learning about people and their accomplishments in a more in-depth way, beyond knowing a person's name and about their family. Professionals at the Quincy Senior and Family Supportive Living Residence, in Quincy, IL, developed an approach in which staff interviewed residents to find out what five accomplishments they were most proud of over their lifetimes. These five accomplishments were then published in a monthly newsletter, anonymously, and other residents tried to guess who they were by the clues provided (Illinois Pioneer Coalition, 2010). This same facility has three other programs designed to foster relationships, support resident involvement, and create community, including in-service programs, resident-centered hospice services, and a cocktail hour.

The in-service program provides educational programs for staff that includes residents. Residents have the opportunity to participate in sessions and to contribute their experiences as input. An example of the type of in-service includes such topics as "Signs and Symptoms of Diabetes," and "Managing Your Cholesterol," as well as other common health conditions.

The resident-centered hospice program was developed in response to those residents who do not have family available to sit with them, especially during the night, in their last life's journey. Volunteers from the residents living within this specific facility share the shifts to help families or people who have no family support.

The last program is focused around a happy hour concept, the purpose of which is to help build relationships among staff, families, and residents. Many residents have no family or outside social connections, so the concept of a happy hour, complete with beverages (adult and otherwise), hors d'oeurves, and opportunities for sharing has been a strategy to help people mingle, learn about the lives of others within the home, and to build community and relationships.

A Girl Scout activity that began as an activity to expose young women to elders living in a long-term care facility in Creve Coeur, MO, blossomed into a wonderful web of connectedness for the young scouts, their families, and residents. The members of the troop were assigned residents, and each scout learned about one person's life highlights through some structured interview questions. The girls followed up by developing either a storyboard frame or scrapbook, and then shared it with the resident, the troop, and other individuals in the facility. Feedback from young and old was overwhelmingly positive, and many long-term relationships blossomed. One girl went to the family home of one of the residents and took pictures of the home as part of her scrapbook that she left the resident. Although this began as a simple exercise, the outcome blossomed into an ongoing project that became an intergenerational building of community connections within the facility and between the Girl Scout troop and the facility (personal communication, Linda Pipes, July 5, 2011).

This section showcased the importance of family and community engagement, along with some examples of strategies that have been used to foster these relationships. Intertwined with building supports between families and communities is the understanding of the linkage between social supports and well-being, and the role this linkage plays.

THE LINKAGE BETWEEN SOCIAL SUPPORTS AND WELL-BEING

It is no surprise that people residing within long-term care settings are more frail than older adults living in the community. In general, their functional status and physical abilities are more limited. As one ages, one becomes more vulnerable to a decline in physical functioning. Functional disability has been shown to affect the subjective well-being of the individual and has been associated with increased morbidity and mortality. Social support is commonly assumed to protect people from the experience of psychological distress and to enhance well-being (Blazer, 2008). Fiksenbaum, Greenglass, Marques, and Eaton (2005) found that the lower the functional ability of an older adult (61 years and older), the more satisfaction there was with extensions of social support. They also found that people who were more incapacitated were more likely to suffer from depression; thus, social support is an important and powerful resource for people with limited capacities.

Lang and Schutze (2002) examined social support and older people's subjective well-being among a sample of German families. They focused on adult children's supportive behaviors toward their parents. Parents were most satisfied with their adult children when children provided affection and emotional support. They did not perceive support, however, when their children challenged their autonomy. The findings also suggest that filial autonomy may facilitate supportive behaviors that contribute to older parents' social-emotional needs (Friedemann, Montgomery, Mailberger, & Smith, 2007; Lang & Schutze, 2002).

Owusu-Ansah (2008) added to Lang and Schutze's (2002) findings and suggested that the essential "ingredients" for psychological and subjective well-being include enjoyment of good health, some financial stability, meaningful ties with others, a sense of purpose and direction in life, the ability to manage complex life demands, a healthy self-acceptance, and a commitment to personal development. Extending these findings into long-term care settings suggests that older adults' well-being would be tied to social connections and valuation of the contributions people had made throughout their lives, despite their current frailties. Ashida and Heaney (2008) found that frequent contact with social network members was positively associated with social support, and perceived social connectedness was positively associated with one's health status. Efforts to enhance older adults' social relationships can be focused on developing friends and companions, allowing them to feel socially engaged and thus reinforcing the value of social connection, family, and community for older adults in long-term care settings.

Bowling (2011) added to the importance of social support by exploring factors that contribute to overall well-being for older adults. Bowling found that self-rated health, mental health symptoms, long-standing illness, and social support were all factors that led to overall well-being; however, social support was the main contributing factor.

Some experts have suggested that social isolation in older people is a growing public health concern within community and continuing care settings, especially in light of the growing proportion of older people in the U.S. population. Social isolation is prevalent among older people, and evidence indicates the detrimental effect it can have on health and well-being. Dickens, Richards, Grieves, and Campbell (2011) carried out a meta-analysis of studies to identify and assess the effectiveness of interventions designed to alleviate social isolation and loneliness in older people. They found that the common characteristics of effective interventions were that they offered social activity and/or support within a group format and had been developed on the basis of some theoretical foundations. Interventions in which older people are active participants also appeared more likely to be effective. Dickens et al.'s review further substantiates the importance of social connections with family and community in efforts to help people living in long-term care facilities remain mentally vital and maintain their sense of well-being.

In the preceding section, readers were introduced to some strategies to create community and social connections in long-term care facilities for older adults through intergenerational programs. Li, Fok, and Fung (2011) explored how these intergenerational relationships influenced older adults' well-being and satisfaction and found that, in fact, the process of reciprocity between generations was of benefit to both parties. The results of their study of 107 older adults and 96 young adults revealed that the social interactions had more benefits for the older adults, created a higher sense of well-being for the older adults, and contributed to a higher degree of life satisfaction than the younger adults. However, the younger adults reported that the relationships were helpful in understanding people outside their peer group and in building interpersonal characteristics with the older adults. Given that the younger cohort had more social outlets on which to rely, it was no surprise that the older adult group would find the relationships more nurturing than the younger cohort; however, the study continues to support the importance of social support and the contributions that social connections make to older adults. Li et al.'s findings support those of Lou (2010), who explored the role of social support from grandchildren in a Chinese sample of elders and their grandchildren and found that emotional support from grandchildren was a major contributing factor to the well-being of their grandparents.

Up to now, the concepts of social support and well-being have been explored, but there is also a link between well-being and vulnerability to mistreatment of elders. Luo and Waite (2011) explored the role of social support and psychological well-being in mistreatment. In their sample of nearly 3,000 older adults ranging in age from 57 to 85, they found that people who experienced lower levels of positive support, higher levels of criticism from close relationships, and feelings of social isolation were more likely to report mistreatment experiences. They concluded that older adults with fewer psychosocial resources and fewer opportunities for social support and social connections with family and community seem to be more vulnerable to mistreatment and more likely to have a lower level of overall well-being. This concept appears to be important for older adults aging in place (Gardner, 2011); for helping older adults maintain the sense of control and autonomy in their lives (Ferguson & Goodwin, 2010); and for maintaining well-being in the face of chronic health conditions (Anaby, Miller, Eng, Jarus, & Noreau, 2011), including type 2 diabetes (Gallegos-Carrillo, García-Peña, Durán-Muñoz, Flores, & Salmerón, 2009).

Thus far, this section has discussed the role of social support and well-being, but a question remains: Does well-being depend on specific strategies within one's social relationships with others? To explore this question, Merz and Huxhold (2010) compared different types and providers of support to older adults. Their research team paid attention to the differences between well-being associated with kin and non-kin providers and with emotional support and instrumental support. They found that people with high-quality relationships who received instrumental support (help with activities of daily living) from kin did not experience decreased well-being. When the relationship with a family carer or supporter is characterized by high quality, the challenges of frailties in old age, such as decreasing capacities and an increasing need for social support, can be met without compromising one's well-being.

The next section of this chapter reviews the specific benchmarks within the ACCT and explores how to integrate these benchmarks into practice.

FAMILY AND COMMUNITY BENCHMARKS

Thus far we have reviewed the literature on the relationship between social supports, connections, and well-being. In addition, we have explored examples of family and community connections and been enlightened on how these connections have an impact on the lives of older adults. In this section, we will review some of the benchmarks identified by the ACCT and explore how to integrate these benchmarks into practice.

Intergenerational Relationships

Benchmark: The facility has an intergenerational program in which children customarily interact with residents at least once a week.

Intergenerational activities have a positive impact on people—that is, older adults and the younger generation. Although these types of relationships can be facilitated through a variety of strategies, the culture change paradigm has established a benchmark that facilities have an intergenerational program in which children customarily interact with residents at least once a week. The benefits to residents have been found to be multifaceted and include lowered agitation levels for residents (Ward, Kamp, & Newman, 1996; Pilkington, 2012).

Several strategies can be used to promote intergenerational activities. One popular idea is to have on-site child day care centers where residents are involved. The Fairport Baptist Home in Fairport, NY; Providence Mt. St. Vincent, Springfield, MA; Teresian House, Albany, NY and Evergreen Retirement Community, OshGosh, Wisconsin, all have these on-site day care approaches. Within these day care centers the amount of intergenerational involvement can vary; however, children and older adults can participate daily in activities together, through reading, cooking, artwork, and meal/snack time (Hammarström & Torres, 2012).

Brookhaven Center, in Findley, OH, has designed a model of child day care that takes place within the household model of care. The environment was built with input from residents, which resulted in a "family living space" with comfortable seating and tables used by adults and children sitting side by side (Norton, 2006).

Other strategies to promote intergenerational programming can include service learning projects between high school students and homes. Students can engage in various types of interviewing projects or oral history projects with residents. Girl Scout and Boy Scout troops can also involve residents in local homes with oral history projects. Students can also benefit from health history projects by working with older adults to identify health conditions they have or may have had and then search the Internet with them to find information about this condition. This type of exercise helps the younger generation learn about health issues that older adults may experience and helps build health literacy for the older adult.

Sunny Home Nursing Center of Joliet, IL, has planned an annual 3-day summer camp jointly with the Joliet Park District as a strategy to facilitate intergenerational relationships. Activities include crafts, games, music, and dance. Participants range in age from 3 to 94 and the number of children who attend annually can range from 100 to 170 (Illinois Pioneer Coalition, 2010).

This benchmark appears to be one that is easily attainable. In a recent report published by the Pioneer Network, of a sample of 319 facilities, 181 (56.7%) surveyed across the United States and Canada had partially implemented this benchmark (Pioneer Network, 2011).

Meeting Space

Benchmark: The facility makes space available for community groups to meet, with residents welcome to attend.

According to this benchmark, facilities would make space available for community groups to meet in the facility, with residents welcome to attend. I myself have experienced this approach in several ways. For several years running, I have held a graduate-level class entitled "Mental Health and Aging" at a local assisted-living facility. Weekly class topics are announced to the residents through flyers and bulletin board postings. Residents are welcome to attend. The feedback has been exceptionally positive. Residents value the opportunity to learn theoretical concepts behind their experiences, and students value the opportunity to discuss concepts with elders and gain knowledge not only from the literature but also from first-hand experience. Students will often bring their children with them, which gives this younger generation a chance to interact with older residents.

A second example of holding group meetings in a long-term care facility is a facility that hosted meetings of the local League of Women Voters group in the community room. Older women enjoy the opportunity to meet with their younger peers and stay involved in civic matters. The relationships built between the group and the facility also made it possible to host a "candidate tea" with local candidates running in state and local elections.

A third example of shared meeting space with the community can be found in Shell Point Retirement Community in Fort Meyers, FL. The retirement community hosts a number of "lifelong learning" speakers and sells tickets for community members to attend. This approach is also used as a fundraiser for the retirement community, but it benefits both the retirement community and the broader community.

This benchmark appears to be easily attainable. In a recent report published by the Pioneer Network (2011), of a sample of 319 facilities, 216 (67.7%) across the United States and Canada surveyed had implemented this benchmark.

Guest Rooms

> Benchmark: Private guest rooms are available for visitors at no or minimal cost for overnight stays.

Ideally, facilities would have private guest rooms available for visitors at no or minimal cost for overnight stays, which forms the basis for this benchmark. Guest rooms provide the opportunity for family members to visit, especially family members traveling from a distance. Shell Point Village provides for guests of residents by making rooms available for use by residents and their family members during short-term stays. This has proven to be a popular opportunity, especially during the tourist season for those wanting to vacation and visit family members.

Teresian House and Providence Mt. St. Vincent also have guest rooms. Teresian House reports that the guest rooms are used by families who travel from a distance as well as by families of residents who are passing through the last stage of their life journey. Although a nominal fee is charged for the use of the room and meals, the fee is a fraction of a hotel stay, although I was not able to determine the actual costs. In addition to family visits within the guest room, family parties also can be held in the community room and private dining rooms.

Food/Entertainment Provisions

> *Benchmark: The facility has a café/restaurant/tavern/canteen available to residents, families, and visitors at which residents and family can purchase food and drinks.*

Most facilities have some provision for entertainment, but this may be intermittent. To meet this benchmark, a facility will have a café/restaurant/tavern/canteen available to residents, families, and visitors at which they can purchase food and drinks.

Shalom Village in Overland Park, KS, has a kosher café that is open to residents, families, staff, and the general public. This facility meets the needs not only of residents but also of the broader community.

Some facilities have developed a look of a "downtown, small town" with a frontage that makes the facility appear to be part of a larger community, and some offer places for residents to sit with their family while providing some privacy. An example of this is the Main Street Café in a midwestern facility, as illustrated in Figure 7.1.

An example of the positive impact of this benchmark can be summed up in the case of Sophia. Sophia enjoys having her brothers and sisters-in-law visit her home. The men often will go to the "Tavern" while the women enjoy a cup of tea in the café. Sophia feels that if it is not possible for her to travel outside her facility due to her mobility needs, then the next best thing is to go to "the main strip." Sometimes, local community groups also come and provide entertainment in the Tavern.

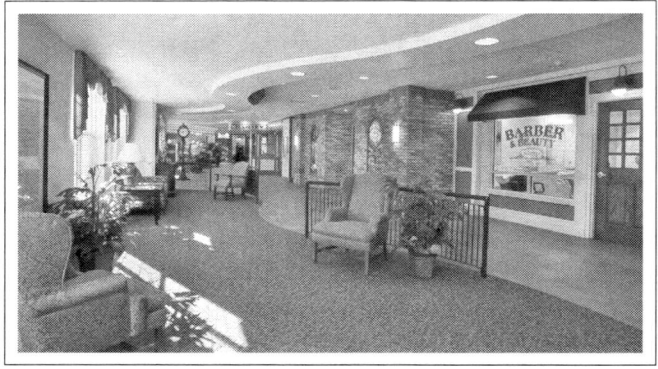

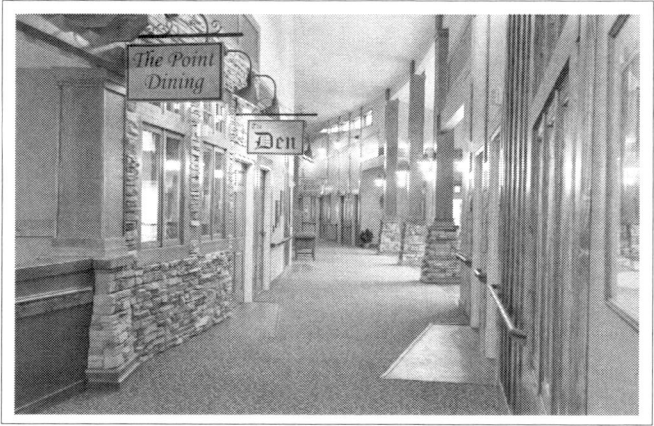

FIGURE 7.1 Café Suite Designed with a "Downtown" Small Town Touch
Source: Horty Elving Architectural Group.

Dining Areas

Benchmark: The facility has a special dining room available for family use/gatherings that is separate from regular dining areas.

It is anticipated that if a facility is to meet this benchmark, a special dining room will be available for family use/gatherings that is separate from the regular dining areas. Long-term care facilities often have private dining rooms available that family members can book for a meal, party, or family gathering. Private dining rooms or spaces take on many different looks, but they all have one feature in common: They provide privacy and comfort when family or friends visit. Some facilities will cater dinner for a resident, whereas others provide dishes and

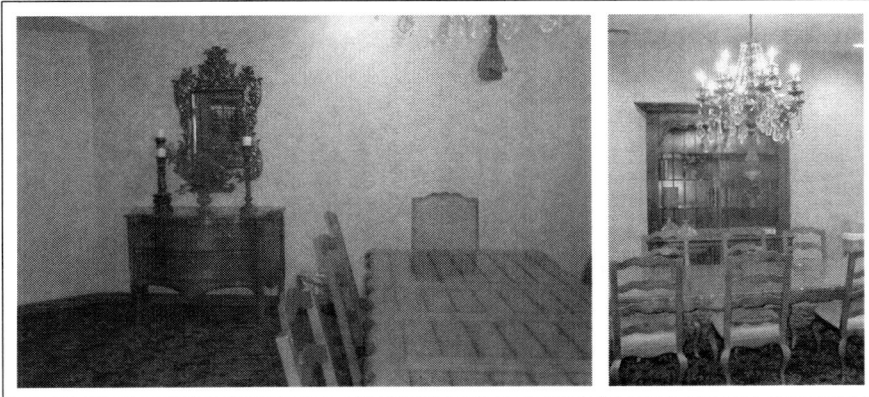

FIGURE 7.2 Private Dining Room

Source: Tuscany Village and Rehabilitation Center.

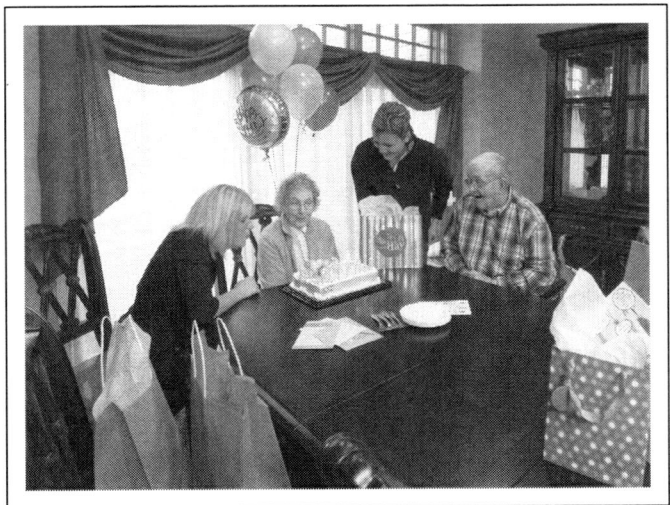

FIGURE 7.3 Private Dining Room and Birthday Party Celebration

Source: Horty Elving Architectural Group.

everything needed for a catered meal. Residents with large extended families enjoy these privileges and feel that they are still able to entertain their loved ones. Figures 7.2 and 7.3 provide two illustrations of a private dining room option.

For example, Ann and her family enjoyed her 87th birthday celebration while she was in rehabilitation during her short stay in residence. The family brought in a cake for dessert and the facility provided a small home-style buffet dinner for the family, all served in the facility/home dining room areas.

This benchmark appears to be easily attainable. In a recent report published by the Pioneer Network (2011), of a sample of 319 facilities across the United States and Canada, 227 (71.2%) had implemented this benchmark.

Kitchen Facilities

> Benchmark: A kitchenette or kitchen area with, at a minimum, a refrigerator and stove, where cooking and baking are encouraged, is available to families, residents, and staff.

Kitchen facilities are an important dimension of family life. This benchmark strives to ensure that facilities will have a kitchenette or kitchen area with, at a minimum, a refrigerator and stove available to families, residents, and staff, where cooking and baking are encouraged.

Household models with full kitchen facilities tend to make these available to their residents, family, and staff (Norton, 2006). Elders are generally elated when asked to prepare a favorite recipe for friends or share meals with family members (Bump, 2005). My own students experienced this firsthand through one of our classroom field trips to a regional facility known for exercising the culture change paradigm. We had agreed to meet for a potluck lunch, and the students all brought a dish to share. Much to our surprise, the residents had also prepared an elaborate spread. During our discussion, one of the students, impressed with the oatmeal chocolate chip raisin cookies that had been prepared, commented on them, and complimented how tasty they were. Within seconds, one of the wheelchair-bound residents announced with great pride that she had prepared them for our visit, and it was one of her favorite family recipes. Within minutes, she located the recipe within the recipe file of the household kitchen and, with the help of a certified nursing assistant, provided a copy of the recipe to each of the students in our group.

SUMMARY

This chapter addressed strategies and benchmarks to enhance family and community involvement within long-term care settings. The chapter began with a review of the importance of social supports on people's functioning and adaptation. Throughout the chapter, benchmarks to help facilities embrace a culture change paradigm within long-term care settings were reviewed, and strategies to address these benchmarks were discussed.

DISCUSSION/REFLECTION QUESTIONS

1. Consider the benchmarks presented throughout this chapter. Identify three specific benchmark items that you would not have thought of prior to reading the chapter. How do these benchmarks integrate one's family and community involvement to be more in line with a culture change paradigm?
2. Identify three benchmarks within the family/community practice domain that you feel have been met within facilities that you either worked in or have been exposed to. Explain why you feel these benchmarks were met.
3. Identify three strategies that you and your team could use to address at least one (or up to three) specific benchmarks in the family and community practice domain.
4. Think about a service learning project you and your classmates or colleagues could get involved in to help a local facility (or the facility in which you currently work) to help meet one of the benchmarks in the family and community practice domain. What steps will you need to put into place to accomplish this goal?

REFERENCES

Anaby, D., Miller, W., Eng, J., Jarus, T., & Noreau, L. (2011). Participation and well-being among older adults living with chronic conditions. *Social Indicators Research, 100,* 171–183.

Andonian, L., & MacRae, A. (2011). Well older adults within an urban context: Strategies to create and maintain social participation. *British Journal of Occupational Therapy, 74,* 2–11.

Ashida, S., & Heaney, C. A. (2008). Differential associations of social support and social connectedness with structural features of social networks and the health status of older adults. *Journal of Aging and Health, 20,* 872–893.

Blazer, D. G. (2008). How do you feel about . . . ? Health outcomes in late life and self perceptions of health and well-being. *The Gerontologist, 48,* 415–422.

Bowling, A. (2011). Do older and younger people differ in their reported well-being? A national survey of adults in Britain. *Family Practice, 28,* 145–155.

Bump, L. (2005). The process of physical design: Regulations and the physical design. *Culture Change Now, 3,* 10–17.

Cheng, S., Li, K., Leung, E. M. F., & Chan, C. M. (2011). Social exchanges and subjective well being: Do sources of positive and negative exchanges matter? *Journals of Gerontology: Series B: Psychological Sciences and Social Sciences, 66,* 708–718.

Dickens, A. P., Richards, S. H., Greaves, C. J., & Campbell, J. L. (2011). Interventions targeting social isolation in older people: A systematic review. *BMC Public Health, 11,* 647.

Fiksenbaum, L. M., Greenglass, E. R., Marques, S. R., & Eaton, J. (2005). A psychosocial model of functional disability. *Ageing International, 30,* 278–295.

Ferguson, S. J., & Goodwin, A. D. (2010). Optimism and well-being in older adults: The mediating role of social support and perceived control. *International Journal of Aging and Human Development, 71*, 43–68.
Friedemann, M. L., Montgomery, R. J., Mailberger, B., & Smith, A. A. (2007). Family involvement in the nursing home: Family oriented practices and staff–family relationships. *Research in Nursing and Health, 20*, 527–537.
Gallegos-Carrillo, K., García-Peña, C., Durán-Muñoz, C. A., Flores, Y. N., & Salmerón, J. (2009). Relationship between social support and the physical and mental wellbeing of older Mexican adults with diabetes. *Revista de Investigación Clínica, 61*, 383–391.
Gardner, P. J. (2011). Natural neighborhood networks—Important social networks in the lives of older adults aging in place. *Journal of Aging Studies, 25* (3), 263–271.
Hammarström, G., & Torres, S. (2012). Variations in subjective well-being when "aging in place"—A matter of acceptance, predictability and control. *Journal of Aging Studies, 26*, 192–203.
Illinois Pioneer Coalition. (2010). *Tales from the prairie: Culture change practices in Illinois long term care communities*. Quincy: Author.
Lang, F., & Schutze, Y. (2002). Adult children's supportive behaviors and older parents' subjective well-being: A developmental perspective on intergenerational relationships. *Journal of Social Issues, 58*, 661–680.
Li, T., Fok, H. K., & Fung, H. H. (2011). Is reciprocity always beneficial? Age differences in the association between support balance and life satisfaction. *Aging & Mental Health, 15*, 541–547.
Lou, V. (2010). Life satisfaction of older adults in Hong Kong: The role of social support from grandchildren. *Social Indicators Research, 95*, 377–391.
Luo, Y., & Waite, L. (2011). Mistreatment and psychological well-being among older adults: Exploring the role of psychosocial resources and deficits. *Journals of Gerontology: Series B: Psychological Sciences and Social Sciences, 66B*, 217–229.
Merz, E., & Huxhold, O. (2010). Well-being depends on social relationship characteristics: Comparing different types and providers of support to older adults. *Ageing & Society, 30*, 843–857.
Norton, L. (2006). *A tale of transformation: Four stages to tell a story*. Washington, DC: American Health Quality Foundation.
Owusu-Ansah, F. E. (2008). Control perceptions and control appraisal: Relation to measures of subjective well-being. *Ghana Medical Journal, 42*, 61–67.
Pilkington, P. D., Windsor, T., & Crisp, D. A. (2012). Volunteering and subjective well-being in midlife and older adults: The role of supportive social networks. *Journals of Gerontology: Series B: Psychological Sciences and Social Sciences, 67B*, 249–260.
Pioneer Network. (2011). *Artifacts of Culture Change benchmark reports, 04/01/2010 3/31/2011*. Retrieved from http://www.artifactsofculturechange.org/Data/Documents/Tools%20for%20Change-Artifacts%20v3.pdf
Schoeneman, K., & Bowman, C. (2006). *Development of the Artifacts of Culture Change Tool: Report of Contract HHSM-500-2005-00076P (Technical report)*. Baltimore, MD: Centers for Medicaid & Medicare Services. Retrieved from http://www.artifactsofculturechange.org/Data/Documents/artifacts.pdf
Ward, C., Kamp, L., & Newman, S. (1999). Activities. *Adaptations and Aging Journal, 20*, 61–76.

8

Leadership Benchmarks/ Artifacts

Leadership practices can influence the heart and soul of how long-term care facilities deliver support to elderly people and people with disabilities and how polices/practices are actually implemented. These practices form the basis on which many residents and their families define quality or satisfaction. This chapter identifies and discusses the leadership benchmarks identified in the Artifacts for Culture Change Assessment Tool (ACCT; Schoeneman & Bowman, 2006) and provides ideas how some of them can be executed within the culture change paradigm. Examples from successful facilities are offered to provide readers with an understanding of how leadership practices can play a role in the development of a culture change paradigm.

DEFINING LEADERSHIP

The term *leadership* has been explored for centuries, and the concept of leadership has spanned managers, dictators, facilitators, and orchestrators. The examination of leadership has taken on a variety of twists and turns over time, including explorations of leadership as task oriented and as person centered (Allen, 2008; Rakich, Longest, & Darr, 1995; Stodgill, 1974; Tannenbaum & Schmidt, 1973; Vroom & Jago, 1988). Management theories have explored and have linked effective leadership with competent management or charisma (Conger & Kanungo, 1988), and transformational leadership strategies (Rakich, Longest, & Darr, 1992). Advocates of servant leadership (Greenleaf, 1998) propose that leaders must serve their constituents and differentiate this leadership style from others that are more directive, or top-down, in orientation.

Kouzes and Posner (1987) defined leadership as a combination of five specific practices that, when integrated as a whole, help people showcase and perform at their very best. These authors argued against leadership as a top-down concept. They claimed that leadership exists throughout an organization and that change is facilitated throughout the organization by means of leadership practices. Kouzes and Posner also suggested that leadership is an interactive process that occurs throughout all levels of the organization. This philosophy lends itself well to the culture change paradigm, because much of the efforts within organizations to change the culture of facilities does not take place from the top down but probably from the trenches on up! With this approach, it becomes more feasible to see and recognize organizational change.

The five leadership practices Kouzes and Posner (1987) identified include (a) Modeling the Way, (b) Inspiring a Shared Vision, (c) Challenging the Process, (d) Enabling Others to Act, and (e) Encouraging the Heart. These practices evolved in the mid-1980s after the publication of a detailed compilation of stories that Kouzes and Posner collected during their work with Fortune 500 companies as they tried to identify how people defined their personal best as a leader. A detailed factor analysis of the stories led to a model that comprises the five factors and 30 variables or activities associated with each of the five factors. These can be found in an instrument known as the Leadership Practices Inventory (2012), or in books written by Kouzes and Posner (2012). The specific practices identified through the five leadership practices are described further in the following.

In the leadership practice titled "Modeling the Way," leaders establish principles concerning the way people (constituents, peers, colleagues, and customers alike) should be treated and the way goals should be pursued (Kouzes & Posner, 1987). They create standards of excellence and then set an example for others to follow. Because the prospect of complex change can overwhelm people and stifle action, leaders set interim goals so that people can achieve small wins as they work toward larger objectives. These leaders (staff) unravel bureaucracy when it impedes action, they put up signposts when people are unsure of where to go or how to get there, and they create opportunities for victory. Within long-term care settings, these practices can be executed through establishing standards of care and practice, using person-centered care benchmarks. Staff can work toward specific goals that they have established or identified with their team members.

The second leadership practice, "Inspiring a Shared Vision," implies that people throughout organizations have the ability to inspire a shared vision. These leaders are passionate about the reality and their perception that they can make a difference. They see the future, create a vision for what they believe can be the ideal, and enlist the support from others. Notably, their quiet persuasion or their charisma and dynamic nature help them enlist others in the dream or goal. The concept of inspiring a shared vision breathes life into their visions and engages people to visualize exciting options and opportunities for the future.

The concept of "Challenging the Process" pushes people to seek opportunities to change the status quo and thus reshape the current practices. Leaders who exercise this practice are constantly on the lookout for ways to improve their organization, especially through risk taking and innovation. Inherent in taking risks is the possibility of making mistakes and failing. Because leaders know that risk taking involves mistakes and failures, they accept the inevitable disappointments as learning opportunities.

Kouzes and Posner's (1987) fourth area of leadership practice is known as "Enabling Others to Act." Effective leadership includes collaborations and teams that are filled with energy, drive, and enthusiasm. Through this process, others get engaged and become involved. Mutual respect creates personhood, no matter what role the person may be in, from facility resident to CEO/president. Effective leaders who enable others to act know how to create an atmosphere of trust and human dignity, and through the process are able to provide strength and the belief that each individual is capable and powerful in his or her own right to make a difference in the lives of others.

The last of the five leadership practices is known as "Encouraging the Heart" and relates to nurturing the spirit and social side of one's being. In an effort to sustain hope and determination, individual contributions and small successes need to be nurtured and celebrated on a consistent and regular basis. People feel affirmed, and in return want to contribute, putting their best foot forward. Within the context of a long-term care setting, people at all levels of the organization encourage the heart, from the housekeeping staff to the certified nursing assistant, all the way up the ranks to the administrator.

In summary, leadership can be defined for the purpose of promoting culture change to encompass all levels of the organization and for exercising practices or behaviors that are consistent with modeling the way; inspiring a shared vision; challenging the process; enabling others to act; and encouraging the heart or nurturing others. These components of leadership can easily be translated into long-term care settings.

LEADERSHIP PRACTICES AND PERSON-CENTERED CARE

The leadership practices outlined by Kouzes and Posner (1987) mesh well with an approach to person-centered care. Generally speaking, the directors of nursing and administrators, two key roles that are perceived to traditionally provide leadership within long-term care or continuing care settings, probably would embrace the leadership practices outlined by Kouzes and Posner (2012); however, all levels of stakeholders within the organization will probably be able to participate in some way in a leadership role in efforts to support person-centered care. Certified nursing assistants can easily work toward supporting residents in their choices and needs (enabling others to act) while at the same time encouraging independence when it is being thwarted by family and professionals (challenging the process). The very process of changing the dominant paradigm in facilities will lead to culture change. Kouzes and Posner's later work (2012) has extended the original leadership practices unveiled in earlier works (1987) and extended them into nursing care and long-term care settings.

THE IMPORTANCE OF LEADERSHIP PRACTICES AND PERSON-CENTERED CARE

Kouzes and Posner's (2012) leadership practices play a central role in achieving a person-centered care environment. Each of the practice areas can be implemented by stakeholders throughout the organization, and therefore, within the context of leadership, the process becomes a shared experience. In order for the environment to truly become one that embraces culture change, all must share the same vision. Thus, the practice of *Inspiring a Shared Vision* becomes important for all stakeholders within the system, from the housekeeping staff to the resident council, residents, and so forth, on up to the administrator. As discussed later in this book, the most effective culture change process will take place if it occurs throughout the organization, and from the bottom up, as opposed to from the top down.

The leadership practice of *Modeling the Way* is a central component of showcasing new ways of addressing and partnering with residents to support their care. Staff who embrace traditional practices of care can learn from the role modeling of this specific leadership practice by their peers.

Challenging the Process is a critical leadership component in the effort of moving from specific nursing and residential practices to embracing the culture change paradigm. According to Kouzes and Posner (2012), the six specific practices that align with challenging the process include the following three: (a) seeking out challenging opportunities that test one's skills and abilities, (b) challenging others to try out innovative approaches to their work, and (c) reaching outside the formal boundaries of the continuing care setting to identify new ways to improve the current residential practices. If things do not seem to move in the direction planned, members of the team, who are exercising leadership practices to challenge the process, should ask what they have learned from the situation and seek to improve the outcomes in an effort to move toward a change of culture. Innovators working within the culture change framework who embrace these practices also experiment and take risks to overcome obstacles, even when outcomes are not clearly visible.

Kouzes and Posner's (2012) leadership practice of *Enabling Others to Act* is also important within the context of promoting person-centered care because those who embrace the person-centered care approach can help motivate their peers toward the same goal. Kouzes and Posner found that ways to help enable others to act include developing cooperative relationships among the people with whom one works, treating others with dignity and respect, and actively listening to diverse points of view and supporting the decisions that people make on their own. The process of supporting others' decisions can include both residents and coworkers. Two additional components of this leadership practice include giving people the freedom to decide how to do their work and ensuring that people grow in their jobs by learning new skills and developing themselves.

Encouraging the Heart, the fifth leadership practice Kouzes and Posner (2012) identified, is important in the process of encouraging person-centered care because it promotes and nurtures the individual, in particular, the resident. Leaders who encourage the heart praise others for a job well done and make it a point to let people know about their confidence in others' abilities. Individuals who embrace these leadership attributes also recognize people who exemplify commitment to shared values. *Encouraging the Heart* also creates an enthusiasm that prescribes a certain energy that becomes contagious to all residents and staff. Thus, the well-being of residents improves and their individual autonomy is more likely to be preserved.

This section has attempted to showcase the linkage between leadership practices and person-centered care. The next section explores the linkage among leadership practices, person-centered care, autonomy, and well-being.

THE LINK AMONG LEADERSHIP PRACTICES, PERSON-CENTERED CARE, AUTONOMY, AND WELL-BEING

Successful leadership promotes a healthy workplace and environmental climate. Within the culture change paradigm, leadership also promotes well-being and personal autonomy on the part of residents. Leadership that promotes these values is based on the "modeling the way" and "inspiring a shared vision" styles defined by Kouzes and Posner (2001).

Much of the literature on culture change has focused on care practices or shifts in the environment. To make these changes, however, a shift in leadership practices is paramount. Leadership can occur throughout the organization, though—it is not central to management, especially if one subscribes to Kouzes and Posner's (2012) definition of leadership.

LEADERSHIP PRACTICE BENCHMARKS

This section addresses the leadership practice benchmarks found in the ACCT.

Resident Care Conferences

> Benchmark: Certified nursing assistants (CNAs) attend resident care conferences.

CNAs are generally the individuals within long-term care facilities who have the most direct contact with the residents. From this vantage point, it makes sense that CNAs would have input into the residents' care conferences. This benchmark promotes the attendance of CNAs at resident care conferences and seeks their input.

Resistance to the implementation of this benchmark rests with management, who have voiced the objection that CNAs offer too much information or inappropriate information (Crandall, While, Schuldheis, Amann, & Talerico, 2007). A safeguard against this would be to provide training for CNAs so they can understand what to expect in a care conference, what information is important, and how best to convey the voice and wishes of the resident. However, involvement of the lowest ranking staff within the care practices of residents has been shown to lead to stronger functional outcomes and increased resident and family satisfaction (Caspar, O'Rourke, & Gutman, 2009).

A second issue to consider in the process of implementing CNA participation in care conferences is to examine which paradigm is at play when conducting care conferences. Traditionally, care conferences have been established and conducted within the lens of a medical model paradigm, which makes input from others difficult, especially professionals from the lowest rung on the ladder (i.e., CNAs). This important group of contributors has not been socialized about how and what to contribute to care conferences, which makes their involvement often awkward or token. Using the leadership principles outlined by Kouzes and Posner (2012), along with some training, could enliven the contributions that CNAs make to the overall treatment process.

This benchmark appears to be one that is attainable with some commitment. A recent report published by the Pioneer Network (2011) revealed that, of a sample of 216 facilities across the United States and Canada, over half (126 facilities, 53.3%) indicated they had partially implemented this benchmark.

Family Collaboration

> Benchmark: Residents or family members serve on home quality assessment and assurance committees (e.g., QI, CQI, QA).

The goal of this benchmark of family collaboration is that residents or family members serve on home quality assessment and assurance committees [e.g., quality improvement (QI), continuous quality improvement (CQI), quality assurance committees (QA)].

There is often a resistance on the part of family members to be involved in these committees because they may not feel qualified to make decisions as part of these teams (O'Neil, 2009). A strategy that could help facilitate family involvement might include coaching and mentoring of family members and residents regarding the various roles they can play within facilities and the input they can offer in terms of governance. In return, input should not be regarded as "token" but valued and recognized as important feedback. Family and consumer participation has been linked with improved health outcomes and an overall higher level of consumer satisfaction. Family members can also help interpret a resident's preferences and help the staff understand the value system and lifelong accomplishments that a resident brings to the facility. Unfortunately, all too often family members are seen as adversaries rather than allies in the therapeutic relationship.

This benchmark appears to not be easily attainable. A recent report published by the Pioneer Network (2011) revealed that, of a sample of 216 facilities across the United States and Canada, none had implemented this benchmark.

Buddy Systems

> Benchmark: Residents have an assigned staff member who serves as a "buddy," case coordinator, guardian angel, and so on, to check with the resident regularly and follow up on any concerns. This is in addition to any assigned social services staff.

This benchmark aspires to have residents have an assigned staff member who serves as a buddy, case coordinator, or guardian angel to check with the resident regularly and follow up on any concerns. This should be in addition to any assigned social services staff. The buddy system can also include volunteers at the facility. Volunteers can often be an important bridge between the residents and staff and can follow up on concerns, especially those outside of the realm of an ombudsperson.

In settings where buddy systems were in place, relationships and connections between resident and staff improved, and fewer complaints from the resident or family members ensued (Schoeneman & Bowman, 2006).

Learning Circles

> Benchmark: Learning circles or the equivalent are used regularly in staff and resident meetings in order to give each person adequate time to communicate their perspective.

Learning circles are a specific venue established to facilitate communication. This benchmark seeks that learning circles or their equivalents be used regularly in staff and resident meetings in order to give each person adequate time to share his or her voice and perspective.

What are learning circles, and how can they be implemented? Norton and Verity (2005) described learning circles as follows:

A Learning Circle is a powerful tool for culture change. It is a problem solving tool that helps teams to make decisions and create solutions. The process, when done over several teams, departments and levels provides a way to tap into all of the wisdom of everyone in the organization. Learning Circles ensure that everyone has an opportunity [to] be heard—to provide input and their perspective into decisions and changes being made. Learning Circles should be done with people who are at the level of resident care whenever decisions affecting resident care are being made (p. 50).

Learning circles are used to let everyone within the network—that is, residents, staff, and families—speak. This approach encourages those on the fringe, or those who are quieter, to speak and be heard, and it gives a voice to all in the decision-making process. Many facilities use this technique at least daily to enable people to connect with each other to address concerns and to work through problems (Norton, 2010; Norton & Verity, 2005; Ronch & Weiner, 2003).

Care Meetings/Conferences

Benchmark: Community meetings are held on a regular basis, bringing staff, residents, and families together as a community.

This benchmark strives to hold community meetings on a regular basis, bringing staff, residents, and families together as a community. Barkan (2002) described the experience of promoting community meetings as "a process that challenged their assumptions about what was possible. [Staff] began to act differently, responding to elders in a more individualized way and helping them to make choices" (p. 52). As a result of this process, many of the staff had revived expectations of the elder residents and changed the way they related to the elders (Barkan, 2002).

Community meetings can take the form of forums or informational sessions for the staff, family, and residents only, or in the form of meetings to which members of the broader community are invited. Informational sessions (held with facility members only) could focus on topics related to caregiving or medical issues to help families and loved ones understand the course of a condition or specific disease. Topics on the aging process or specific diagnostic conditions can also be helpful.

Community meetings that incorporate the broader community can include topics of medical interest, caregiving interest, or the aging process. The topics also can be expanded to a range of areas that would entice the broader population. Shell Point Village, located in Fort Myers, FL, offers a regular speaker series that hosts a range of topics, from authors to discussion groups with well-known community personalities. This approach helps build the morale within the institution as well as the community. This approach also helps infuse the facility with new ideas that the staff can incorporate into their roles and management practices.

SUMMARY

This chapter addressed strategies and benchmarks to enhance leadership in efforts to create a homelike approach to long-term care settings. The beginning of the chapter reviewed the importance of leadership and various leadership approaches that can be implemented in long-term care settings. Throughout the chapter, benchmarks to be met in an effort to meet a culture change paradigm within long-term care settings were reviewed, and strategies to address these benchmarks were presented. This chapter is unique in comparison to the other chapters in that leadership is seen as a process in and of itself that can affect the remainder of the movement toward a culture change paradigm.

DISCUSSION/REFLECTION QUESTIONS

1. *Identify two benchmark areas within this chapter that you would not have thought of in an effort to create leadership to be more in line with a culture change paradigm.*
2. *Identify five leadership practices that can affect benchmarks within the leadership domain that you feel have been met within facilities that you either worked in or have been exposed to. Explain why you feel these benchmarks were met.*
3. *Can you identify three strategies that you and your team could use to address at least one (or up to three) specific benchmarks in the leadership domain?*
4. *Think about a service learning project you and your classmates or colleagues could get involved in to help a local facility (or the facility in which you currently work) to help meet one of the benchmarks in the leadership domain. What steps will you need to put into place to accomplish this goal?*

REFERENCES

Allen, J. E. (2008). *Nursing home administration* (5th ed.). New York, NY: Springer Publishing.

Barkan, B. (2002). *The way of the champion: A personal journey, a live oak learner's journal*. Rochester, NY: The Pioneer Network.

Caspar, S., O'Rourke, N., & Gutman, G. M. (2009). The differential influence of culture change models on long-term care staff empowerment and provision of individualized care. *Canadian Journal on Aging, 28*, 165–175.

Conger, J. A., & Kanungo, R. (1988). *Charismatic leadership: The elusive factor in organizations*. San Francisco, CA: Jossey-Bass.

Crandall, L. G., White, D. L., Schuldheis, S., & Talerico, K. A. (2007). Initiating person centered care practices in long-term care facilities. *Journal of Gerontological Nursing, 33*(11), 47–56

Greenleaf, R. (1998). *The power of servant leadership*. San Francisco, CA: Berret-Koehler.

Kouzes, J., & Posner, B. (1987). *The leadership challenge: How to get extraordinary things done in organizations*. San Francisco, CA: Jossey-Bass.

Kouzes, J., & Posner, B. (2001). *The leadership practices inventory—online version*. San Francisco, CA: Wiley Retrieved from http://consummatecoaching.com/images/LPI-WB_book.pdf

Kouzes J., & Posner, B. (2012). *The leadership challenge: How to get extraordinary things in organizations* (5th ed.). San Francisco, CA: Wiley.

Norton, E. S. (2010). Sustaining a person-centered care environment. *Long-Term Living: For the Continuing Care Professional, 59*(8), 40–42.

Norton, L., & Verity, J. (2005). *The learning circle process*. Dementia Care Australia. Retrieved from http://www.dhs.wisconsin.gov/aging/genage/Pubs/LearningCircleGuide.pdf

O'Neil, T. (2009). Adding families to the care team. Family members hold keys to person-centered care. *Health Progress, 90*(6), 48–50.

Pioneer Network. (2011). *Artifacts of culture change benchmark reports, 04/01/2010–3/31/2011*. Retrieved from www.artifactsofculturechange.org

Rakich, J., Longest, B. B., & Darr, K. (1995). *Managing health services organizations*. Baltimore, MD: Health Professions Press.

Ronch, J. & Weiner, A. (2003). Culture change in long term care. New York, NY: Haworth Press.

Schoeneman, K., & Bowman, C. (2006). *Development of the artifacts of culture change tool: Report of Contract HHSM-500-2005-00076P* (Technical report). Baltimore, MD: Centers for Medicaid & Medicare Services. Retrieved from http://www.artifactsofculturechange.org/Data/Documents/artifacts.pdf

Stodgill, R. M. (1974). *Handbook of leadership: A survey of the literature*. New York, NY: Free Press.

Tannenbaum, R., & Schmidt, W. H. (1973). How to choose a leadership pattern. *Harvard Business Review, 51*, 162–180.

Vroom, V. H., & Jago, A. G. (1988). *The new leadership: Managing participation in organizations*. Englewood Cliffs, NJ: Prentice Hall.

9

Workplace Practice Benchmarks/Artifacts

WORKPLACE PRACTICES AND PERSON-CENTERED CARE

Workplace practices, policies, and culture will influence the performance of employees and workers, as well as the overall general care outcomes in long-term care facilities. These various elements also will affect how residents and family members perceive their experiences within the facility. This chapter examines the workplace practices identified as benchmarks in the Artifacts for Culture Change Tool (ACCT) and discusses ideas about how some of them can be executed within the culture change paradigm. Examples from successful facilities are described to facilitate reader comprehension of the care practices being discussed.

THE IMPORTANCE OF WORKPLACE PRACTICES AND PERSON-CENTERED CARE

Workplace practices play a significant role in the development and sustainability of a culture change environment. The two are linked to employee turnover and employee satisfaction. Eaton (2000) found that caregivers working within a culture in which they were respected and valued tended to be more satisfied, and observed that these settings experienced lower employee turnover. Flesner (2003) expounded on these findings and examined a series of nursing homes that had embraced the culture change philosophy. She found that staff turnover was lower than that in traditional nursing homes and that a waiting list for staff positions also existed. In other words, people were lining up waiting to be able to secure jobs in facilities that had embraced a culture change philosophy or that had developed a culture that respected a person-centered care philosophy. Employees embraced the idea that they were able to form meaningful and long-lasting relationships with the residents when working within a person-centered care facility. They also looked forward to coming to work and contributing to the overall well-being of the residents (Flesner, 2003).

THE LINK AMONG WORKPLACE PRACTICES, PERSON-CENTERED CARE, AUTONOMY, AND WELL-BEING

Workplace practices play a role in the overall well-being of both residents and staff, and serve as the foundation for person-centered care and overall autonomy (Tellis-Nayak, 2007). Outcomes from Tellis-Nayak's (2007) research provide empirical support for the role positive workplace practices play in both the workplace culture and well-being of individual residents. Norton (2010) encouraged the sustaining of a person-centered environment because of the strong relationship it has with individual autonomy and well-being for both staff and residents.

WORKPLACE PRACTICE BENCHMARKS

Nursing Staff—Registered Nurses

Benchmark: Registered nurses (RNs) consistently work with the residents of the same neighborhood/household/unit, with no rotation.

The first benchmark within this domain suggests that RNs should consistently work with the residents of the same neighborhood/household/unit, with no rotation.

Eaton (2001) found that nurses enjoyed consistent patient contact and with his sample, he found that 95% of nurses did not like to move around from unit to unit. Working with the same resident led to some important shifts for both the staff and residents. Residents, formerly perceived as being needy and demanding, became much more compliant because their nursing staff became familiar with their particular wants, routines, and behaviors (L. Pedtke, personal communication, June 23, 2012). Staff also found that their roles become more meaningful and interactive between residents and nurses when the latter had consistent assignments because their jobs moved beyond tasks to supporting the resident (L. Pedtke, personal communication, June 23, 2012).

This benchmark appears to be one that is attainable with some commitment to change this policy. A recent report published by the Pioneer Network (2011) revealed that, of a sample of 216 facilities across the United States and Canada over half (140 homes, 64.8%) indicated they had partially implemented this benchmark.

Nursing Staff—Licensed Practical Nurses

Benchmark: Licensed practical nurses (LPNs) consistently work with the residents of the same neighborhood/household/unit, with no rotation.

In addition to having RNs work consistently on the same unit, a second benchmark within this workplace domain calls for LPNs to also consistently work with the residents of the same neighborhood/household/unit, with no rotation. The beauty of consistent assignments is that the elders get to know the staff, and vice versa.

This benchmark appears to be one that is attainable with some commitment to change this policy. A recent report published by the Pioneer Network (2011) revealed that, of a sample of 216 facilities across the United States and Canada, over half (145 facilities, 67.1%) indicated that they had partially implemented this benchmark.

Nursing Staff—Certified Nursing Assistants

Benchmark: Certified nursing assistants (CNAs) consistently work with the residents of the same neighborhood/household/unit, with no rotation.

The third benchmark within this domain suggests that CNAs consistently work with the residents of the same neighborhood/household/unit, with no rotation. Kane et al. (2004) found that this consistency, or permanent assignment to units, was found to be correlated with a higher quality of life. This consistency of caregivers is vitally important for people with dementia and leads to better behavioral outcomes (Barry, 2007; Edvardsson, Fetherstonhaugh, McAuliffe, Nay, & Chenco, 2011). Consistent assignment of staff to units helps lead to a stronger and clearer understanding of the individual resident and his or her specific preferences. If residents feel as if they are understood and that their needs are consistently met, they are more likely to be content and less demanding of staff. Thus, the process of consistent assignments has benefits for both the staff and residents. A less stressful situation can also lead to lower rates of burnout and compassion fatigue.

This benchmark appears to be one that is attainable with some commitment to change. A recent report published by the Pioneer Network (2011) revealed that, of a sample of 216 facilities across the United States and Canada, over half (163 facilities, 75.4%) indicated they had partially implemented this benchmark.

Scheduling

Benchmark: Self-scheduling of work shifts. CNAs develop their own schedule and fill in for absent CNAs. CNAs independently handle the task of scheduling, trading shifts/days, and covering for each other instead of relying on a staffing coordinator.

This benchmark aims to have individual CNAs self-schedule their work shifts. With this approach, CNAs would be responsible for developing their own work schedule and filling in for colleagues who are unable to work or are otherwise absent. Within this approach, CNAs would independently handle the job of scheduling, trading shifts/days, and covering for each other instead of having a staffing coordinator handle this responsibility. The Eden Alternative experience implemented this approach and found that CNAs took their scheduling and backup seriously (Kane, Lum, Cutler, Degenholtz, & Tzy-Chyi, 2007).

This benchmark appears to be one that is attainable with some commitment to change this policy. In the Pioneer Network's (2011) survey of 216 facilities across the United States and Canada, almost all (210 facilities, 97.3%) indicated they had not implemented this benchmark.

This approach may seem too radical for many facilities because of the perception that certain positions should have authority over staffing. Staffing shortages may be of concern, and facilities may not want to risk their reputation by empowering CNA staff in this way; however, there are examples of facilities where this has been accomplished successfully. For example, Eaton (2000) reported that in the first Eden Alternative facility, Chase Memorial in New York, Dr. Bill Thomas asked the nurse aides to make their own schedules, and immediately staff attendance improved as people worked out their responsibilities at home and at work for themselves, rather than having these imposed on them by a supervisor.

Over a decade ago, during the Meeting of Pioneers in Nursing Home Culture Change, Misiorski (1997) reported that the approach with *CNAs doing their own patient assignments as well as their work schedules ... had reduced call outs, they replace[d] themselves, and it benefitted [sic] residents* (cited in Fagan, 1997).

Continuing Education

Benchmark: The facility pays expenses for nonmanagerial staff (e.g., CNAs, direct care nurses) to attend outside conferences/workshops.

This benchmark holds facilities to the standard of paying expenses for nonmanagerial staff, such as CNAs and direct care nurses, to attend outside conferences/workshops. The artifact instrument asks for a "yes" to be checked if at least one nonmanagerial staff member attended an outside conference/workshop paid by the facility in the past year. Continuing education training has continually been perceived as a burdensome expense, especially because it may have involved travel, lodging, and the cost of a workshop. With online training and webinars now more readily available, training opportunities for CNAs are much more accessible.

Continuing education appears to be valued and respected by homes and facilities. A recent report published by the Pioneer Network (2011) revealed that, of a sample of 319 facilities across the United States and Canada, nearly three quarters (255 facilities, 79.9%) indicated they had fully implemented this benchmark.

Uniforms

Benchmark: Staff are not required to wear uniforms or "scrubs."

Staff in homes have traditionally worn "scrubs" within licensed care facilities. Smaller facilities, such as foster care units, have not necessarily followed this standard. Within this benchmark standard, staff would not be required to wear uniforms or scrubs. (As a point of clarification, foster care units are state-approved or licensed homes where a person resides with a "foster" family that provide custodial care. The caretaker is usually paid by a private pay source associated with the resident or by a governmental entity. Foster care with older adults is similar to foster care with children, except the target population differs).

The concept behind this benchmark is to blur the division of roles among the care provider team, so that a team mindset would be easier to foster or develop. Within this approach, everyone, regardless of function (CNA, LPN, or RN), would dress the same way, with only a name badge to differentiate each position.

This benchmark appears to be one that has had a limited degree of support. According to the Pioneer Network's (2011) recent survey of a sample of 319 facilities across the United States and Canada, over three quarters (256 facilities, 80.2%) indicated they had not implemented this benchmark at all.

Cross-Training

Benchmark: The percentage of other staff cross-trained and certified as CNAs in addition to the CNAs in the nursing department.

This benchmark seeks to ensure that other staff are cross-trained and certified as CNAs in addition to the regular CNAs in the nursing department. The rationale behind this benchmark is to enable greater flexibility between aides and nursing assistants and to facilitate aides' helping with the roles of toileting and bathing when residents prefer these roles be undertaken, rather than when the institutional schedule dictates that these duties be performed (Eaton, 2000).

This benchmark appears to be one that is attainable with some commitment. A recent report published by the Pioneer Network (2011) revealed that, of a sample of 319 facilities across the United States and Canada, almost half (147 facilities, 46.8%) indicated they had partially implemented this benchmark.

Activities

Benchmark: Activities, informal or formal, are led by staff in other departments, such as nursing, housekeeping, or others.

This benchmark suggests that activities, informal or formal, are led by staff from other departments, such as nursing and housekeeping. This approach facilitates participation within the care realm of all individuals within a facility. Traditionally, nursing, occupational therapy, physical therapy, and social work professionals have remained within their own professional domains of expertise. Activities developed to reach the entire facility can include these professional groups and expand the reach of the activity workers' duties. An example might be a facility barbeque event. Although organized by the activity director, each of the other professional disciplines takes on the responsibility of participating with different neighborhoods (a term used instead of *wing* or *ward*) to make the event a success. In one instance, the social worker helped staff the refreshment table, and the occupational and physical therapists were responsible for facilitating the games.

This benchmark appears to be one that is attainable per the Pioneer Network's (2011) recent survey: Of 319 facilities across the United States and Canada, nearly two thirds (206 facilities, 65.7%) indicated they had completely implemented this benchmark.

Recognition

> Benchmark: Awards (e.g., Culture Change award, Champion of Change award) are given to staff to recognize commitment to person-directed care. This does not include Employee of the Month awards.

This benchmark challenges facilities to give awards (e.g., Culture Change award, Champion of Change award) to staff who demonstrate a commitment to person-directed care. These do not include Employee of the Month awards. One of the innovative examples of how this can be implemented can be seen through a program known as "Through the Looking Glass," implemented by Aviston Countryside Manor, located in Aviston, IL (Illinois Pioneer Coalition, 2011).

The administrator of Aviston Countryside Manor set up a challenge to staff working throughout the facility to stay at the home as a resident. The individual who stayed the longest (out of four people at a time) would receive a $500 cash prize. The contestants were expected to follow the same rules as residents and were expected to dine with the residents and be cared for by facility staff. As part of the process, each contestant was randomly assigned a series of health conditions and a daily challenge in terms of a behavior. Daily challenges included such things as sitting in a soiled diaper (chocolate pudding served as the proxy for "soiled diaper") to maintaining a liquid diet. Contestants were also faced with a number of dietary challenges that included mechanically processed soft food and problems with chewing. The diagnoses that participating staff members were faced with included congestive heart failure, stroke, left-side paralysis or left-side weakness, and fluid retention. The experience created a strong sensitivity on the part of the workers to the day-to-day challenges the residents faced and the loneliness or isolation that residents may often feel. Overall, this exercise not only heightened sensitivity but also improved staff and resident relationships.

Career Ladders

Benchmark: Career ladder positions are available for CNAs (e.g., CNA II, CNA III, team leader, etc.) so they can hold a position higher than entry level.

This benchmark seeks career ladder positions for CNAs, such as CNA II, CNA III, team leader, and so on, and aspires to give CNAs the opportunity to advance to a position higher than entry level. This helps with job satisfaction and leads to reduced employee turnover.

This benchmark appears to be one that is attainable with some commitment to change this policy. A recent report published by the Pioneer Network (2011) revealed that, of a sample of 319 facilities across the United States and Canada, almost three quarters (235 facilities, 73.6%) indicated they had not implemented this benchmark.

Job Development

Benchmark: A job development program (e.g., CNA to LPN to RN to nurse practitioner) is available to staff.

This benchmark establishes a career path whereby a job development program is available to facilitate staff movement across roles and upward through continuing education. The progression would facilitate the movement from CNA to LPN to RN to nurse practitioner, and so on.

This benchmark appears to be one that is attainable with some commitment toward supporting and encouraging employees to develop professionally. A recent report published by the Pioneer Network (2011) revealed that, of a sample of 319 homes across the United States and Canada, over half (222 facilities, 69.5%) indicated they had fully implemented this benchmark.

Day Care

> Benchmark: On-site day care is available to staff.

Another workplace goal or benchmark includes having day care on site that is available to staff. Research has suggested that a preschool on site has been correlated with a high quality of life (Kane et al., 2004). Day care provides wonderful opportunities for intergenerational programming as well as opportunities for staff to regularly integrate their children into the lives of the older adults with whom they are in contact on a daily basis. The benefits also have an impact on the children, who learn to appreciate the older adult cohort as well. The College of St. Scholastica, located in Duluth, MN, has a continuum-of-care facility located on campus. The residents range from assisted living to skilled nursing care and benefit from the day care participants, as well as college-age students.

Although this benchmark is one that appears to promote quality of life, few facilities have implemented it, according to recent survey results. The Pioneer Network (2011) found, in a sample of 319 facilities across the United States and Canada, that over three quarters (287 facilities, 89.9%) indicated they had not implemented this benchmark.

Volunteer Coordinator

> Benchmark: The facility has an on-staff paid volunteer coordinator in addition to an activity director.

Volunteer coordinators are the lifeblood of many facilities/homes' extracurricular activities. This benchmark asks facilities to have on staff a paid volunteer coordinator in addition to an activity director. It also differentiates between a full-time coordinator (30 hours/week or more), a part-time one (15–30 hours/week), or an unpaid volunteer coordinator.

Employee Evaluations

> Benchmark: Employee evaluations include observable measures of employee support of individual resident choices, control, and preferred routines in all aspects of daily living.

This benchmark suggests that employee evaluations include observable measures of employee support of individual resident choices, control, and preferred routines in all aspects of daily living. If these categories are included on employee evaluations, it will become easier to reward and support employees who demonstrate a commitment to the culture change paradigm.

SUMMARY

This chapter addressed strategies and benchmarks to enhance workplace practices and create a homelike approach to long-term care settings. The first part of the chapter reviewed the importance of workplace practices and the relationship between workplace practices and residential culture. Throughout the chapter, benchmarks to be met in an effort to meet a culture change paradigm within long-term care settings were reviewed, and strategies to address these benchmarks were presented.

DISCUSSION/REFLECTION QUESTIONS

1. *Identify some benchmark areas within this chapter that you would not have thought of in an effort to build workplace policies and practices to be more in line with a culture change paradigm.*
2. *Identify benchmarks within the workplace practice domain that you feel have been met within facilities that you either worked in or have been exposed to. Explain why you feel these benchmarks were met.*
3. *Can you identify three strategies that you and your team could use to address at least one (or up to three) specific benchmarks in the workplace practice domain?*
4. *Take on the role of "administrator" for a week. What policies would you revise within your facility to help meet some of the benchmarks in the workplace domain? What steps will you need to put into place*

to accomplish this goal? Which other stakeholders would you bring to the table to help facilitate your policy changes? What role would these stakeholders have to take on as part of this change process?

REFERENCES

Barry, T. (2007). Nurse aide empowerment strategies and staff stability: Effects on nursing home resident outcomes. *The Gerontologist, 45*, 309–317.

Eaton, S. C. (2000). Beyond unloving care: Making human resource management and patient quality in nursing homes. *International Journal of Human Resource Management, 11*, 591–616.

Eaton, S. (2001). What a difference management makes! Nursing staff turnover variation within a single labor market. In *Report to Congress: Appropriateness of minimum nurse staffing ratios in nursing homes Phase II final report.*

Edvardsson, D., Fetherstonhaugh, D., McAuliffe, L., Nay, R., & Chenco, C. (2011). Satisfaction amongst aged care staff: Exploring the influence of person-centered care provision. *International Psychogeriatrics, 23*, 1205–1212.

Fagan, R. (1997). *Meeting of Pioneers in Nursing Home Culture Change: March 14-16, 1997.* Rochester, NY: Pioneer Network.

Flesner, M. K. (2003). *Person centered care: A model for nursing homes.* (Unpublished doctoral dissertation), University of Missouri—Columbia.

Illinois Pioneer Coalition (2011). *Through the looking glass: Culture change practices in Illinois long term care communities.* Quincy, IL: Author.

Kane, A. R., Pratt, M., Schoeneman, K., Kane, R. L. Bershadsky, B., Cutler, L. J., Giles, K. S., Liu, J., Kang, K., Zhang, L., Kling, K. C., Degenholtz, H. B. (2004). *Measures, indicators, and improvement of quality of life in nursing homes: Final report.* Retrieved from http://www/hpm.umn.edu/ltcResourcesCenter/research/QOL/Final Report to CMS Volume 1.

Kane, R. A., Lum, T., Cutler, L. J., Degenholtz, H. B., & Tzy-Chyi, Y. (2007). Resident outcomes in small-house nursing homes: A longitudinal evaluation of the initial green house program. *Journal of the American Geriatrics Society, 55*, 382–389.

Norton, E. S. (2010). Sustaining a person-centered care environment. *Long-Term Living: For the Continuing Care Professional, 59*(8), 40–42.

Pioneer Network. (2011). *Artifacts of Culture Change benchmark reports, 04/01/2010–3/31/2011.* Retrieved from www.artifactsofculturechange.org.

Tellis-Nayak, V. (2007). A person-centered workplace: The foundation for person-centered caregiving in long-term care. *Journal of the American Medical Directors Association, 8*, 46–54.

10

Outcome Practices

The last category of benchmarks identified in the Artifacts of Culture Change Tool (ACCT; Schoeneman & Bowman, 2006) relates to outcome practices. Although this category of outcome practices seems distant and disconnected from the particular day-to-day care, these items support the array of person-centered care benchmarks. The availability and tenure of staff within a long-term care facility are shaped by outcome practices. The retention of competent and dedicated staff is an important concern for long-term care facilities because, without tenure and continuity, the relationship dimension between staff and residents will be difficult to maintain. This chapter examines the outcome practices identified as benchmarks in the ACCT and suggests ideas as to how some of these areas can be executed within the culture change paradigm. Examples from successful facilities are provided as well.

WHAT ARE OUTCOMES, AND HOW DO THEY RELATE TO IMPROVING PERSON-CENTERED CARE?

Within the context of the ACCT, staffing outcomes are related to the longevity and retention of nursing care staff. Specifically, staffing patterns at the levels of certified nursing assistant (CNA), nursing care staff, director of nursing, and administrator levels are addressed. Adequate staffing patterns ensure that residents are cared for with optimal relationships and that their wants and preferences are respected. In essence, it ensures that person-centered care opportunities are enhanced.

Frequent staff turnover does not facilitate an understanding of the residents or their unique needs and preferences. It also causes distress for the residents, as they grieve the loss of familiar staff and the relationships they have developed with staff.

THE IMPORTANCE OF OUTCOMES

Outcomes—specifically, staffing outcomes—play a central role in the well-being, functional status, and satisfaction of residents in long-term care settings. These concepts have been well articulated in the scientific literature. A recent meta-analysis that examined 713 articles related to quality care, outcomes, and care practices linked the quality of nursing care and stability of nursing care staff with outcomes (Sales et al., 2012). The most frequently cited issues contributing to unsuccessful quality improvement interventions were lack of staff, high staff turnover, and limited time available to train staff in ways that would improve client care. Innovative strategies and supporting research are required to determine how to intervene successfully to improve quality in settings characterized by low staffing levels and predominantly nonprofessional staff. Research on how to effectively enable practitioners to use data to improve quality of care, and ultimately quality of life, needs to be consistently and continually explored to ensure a link between staffing outcomes and quality care.

THE LINK AMONG OUTCOMES, PERSON-CENTERED CARE, AUTONOMY, AND WELL-BEING

At this point, one may ask, "What is the link among outcomes, person-centered care, autonomy, and well-being?" Arling, Kane, Mueller, Bershadsky, and Degenholtz (2007) set out to determine the relationship among nursing home staffing levels, care received by individual residents, and resident quality-related care processes and functional outcomes. In their review of data, nurses recorded resident care time for 5,314 residents on 156 units in 105 facilities in four states (Colorado, Indiana, Minnesota, and Mississippi). The authors linked residents' care times to their measures of health and functioning from minimum data set assessments. Higher overall staffing was associated with more time devoted to direct resident care. The research team also found a connection among nursing home quality, organization, and delivery rather than simply the amount of care available.

Castle and Engberg (2007) examined the influence that staffing levels, turnover, worker stability, and agency staff had on quality of care in nursing homes. They conducted a survey among nursing homes with a sample of 1,071 nursing facilities and focused on the impact of care and quality of life outcomes for residents using a variety of variables, including staff consistency and staff turnover. They found that a variety of staffing characteristics including staffing levels and worker stability, played a role in turnover. They also found a link between worker stability and turnover with quality of life and resident satisfaction; the more stable the workforce, the greater the level of resident satisfaction. Castle and Engberg found that it was not just one dimension that influenced the quality of care and resident satisfaction but rather an interaction among several factors, such as stability in care staff and in leadership (i.e., administrator or director of nursing).

Spilsbury, Hewitt, Stirk, and Bowman (2011) carried out a meta-analysis of studies related to nursing care to explore the relationship between nursing home nurse staffing (proportion of registered nurses [RNs] and support workers) and quality of care for nursing home residents. A focus on numbers of nurses, however, fails to address the influence of other staffing factors (e.g., turnover, agency staff use), training and experience of staff, and care organization and management. "Quality" is a difficult concept to capture directly, and the measures used in the studies of the meta-analysis focused mainly on clinical outcomes for residents. Spilsbury et al.'s systematic mapping review highlights important methodological lessons for future international studies and makes an important contribution to the evidence base of the relationship between the nursing workforce and quality of care and resident outcomes in nursing home settings.

Munn and Zimmerman (2006) studied end-of-life care in long-term care settings to explore the process of the end-of-life experience for family members and residents. In their analysis of nursing homes, they found that adequate staffing, training, and consistency were important to family in a person's last days. "Being there" and being available, along with the way care was delivered, were found to be extremely important in the process of care. Although their study is a bit dated, their findings, based on data from 230 nursing homes and assisted-living facilities, still point to the importance of consistent staffing, staff availability to residents, and the impact these have on people's lives at a time when they are most vulnerable.

In short, the link among outcomes, person-centered care, autonomy, and well-being is central to the comfort and quality of life a person experiences while residing in a long-term care facility. Ensuring that staff are available to residents is important, as is ensuring that the working conditions facilitate staff engagement, and contentment, and desire to continue working in a particular setting. The remainder of this chapter reviews some of the specific outcome benchmarks and describes how they can be implemented in specific facilities.

OUTCOME PRACTICE BENCHMARKS

Longevity of Staff

> Benchmark: What is the average longevity of CNAs?

Average Longevity of CNAs

This benchmark seeks to determine how long CNAs, on average, have been working in a specific home/facility. To compute this number, one would add the number of years each CNA has been employed and then divide that number by the number of CNA staff. For example, the following calculations will help show how to compute this rate for longevity:

CNA Name	Length of Employment
1-Sarah	5 years
2-Linda	2 years
3-Amanda	1 year
4-Kyle	6 months (.5 years)
5-Ticara	7 years
Total = 5 employees	15.5 years

15.5 years divided by 5 employees = 3.1 years rate for longevity of employment for CNA staff.

Ideally, this rate should be computed once per year, but it can also be calculated on a more frequent rate to examine patterns of retention.

Average Longevity of Licensed Practical Nurses (LPNs) in any Position

> Benchmark: What is the average longevity of LPNs?

This benchmark seeks to determine how long LPNs, on average, have been working in a specific home/facility. To compute this number, one would add the number of years each LPN has been employed and then divide that number by the number of LPN staff. For example, the following calculations will help show how to compute this rate for longevity:

LPN Name	Length of Employment
1-Peggy	15 years
2-Lydia	2 years
3-Alicia	8 years
4-Darnell	6 years
5-Latisse	9 months (.75 years)
6-Arwan	4 years
Total = 6 employees	35.75 years

35.75 years divided by 6 employees = 5.9 years

Ideally, this rate should be computed once per year, but it can also be calculated on a more frequent rate to examine patterns of retention.

Average Longevity of RNs/General Nurses (GNs) in any Position

> Benchmark: What is the average longevity of RNs and GNs?

This benchmark seeks to determine how long RNs/GNs, on average, have been working in a specific home/facility. To compute this number, one would add the number of years each RN/GN has been employed and then divide that number by the number of RN/GN staff. For example, the following calculations will help show how to compute this rate for longevity:

RN/GN Name	Length of Employment
1-Melissa	5 years
2-Wendy	22 years
3-Horace	18 months (1.5 years)
4-Bryce	16 years
5-Lavonna	9 years
6-Mary	14 years
7-Shirley	2 years
8-Ashley	1 year
Total = 8 employees	70.5 years 70.5 years divided by 8 employees = 8.8 years

Longevity of the Director of Nursing (in any Position)

> Benchmark: What is the average longevity of the director of nursing?

This benchmark seeks to determine how long the director of nursing, on average, has been working in a specific home/facility. To compute this number, one would add the number of years each director of nursing has been employed, and then divide that number by the number of directors of nursing. The same calculations would be used as in the previous sets of calculations.

Longevity of the Administrator (in any Position)

> Benchmark: What is the average longevity of the administrator?

This benchmark seeks to determine how long the administrator, on average, has been working in a specific home/facility. To compute this number, one would add the number of years each administrator has been employed and then divide that number by the number of administrators. The same calculations would be used as in the previous sets of calculations.

Turnover Rates

> Benchmark: What is the turnover rate for CNAs?

The turnover rate for the number of CNAs would be calculated on the basis of the number who left, voluntarily or involuntarily, in the past 12 months, divided by number of total CNAs employed. Once this is computed, one would find a rate and then assign points on the basis of which percentage level the rate falls under.

For example, Villa Place has 62 CNAs currently employed in its facility. Over the past 12 months, five resigned, and one was involuntarily terminated.

Six (6) left divided by 62 positions.

6/62 = .0967 or 9.6%

Your home's figure ____9.6%____

0–19% (5 points) (on this benchmark, Villa Place would receive 5 points)

20–39% (4 points)

40–59% (3 points)

60–79% (2 points)

80–99% (1 point)

100% and above (0 points)

Turnover Rate for LPNs

Benchmark: What is the turnover rate for LPNs?

The computations for the number of LPNs who left, voluntarily or involuntarily, in the past 12 months, divided by number of total LPNs employed, will be completed in the same way that the figure for the CNAs was computed. The difference is that these figures will be assigned a different point value according to this benchmark because it is more difficult to hire and train LPNs.

Your home's figure _____

0–12% (5 points)

13–25% (4 points)

26–38% (3 points)

39–51% (2 points)

52–65% (1 point)

66 and above (0 points)

Turnover Rate for RNs

Benchmark: What is the turnover rate for RNs?

Once again, the same pattern as in the previous two segments (CNAs and LPNs) will be followed for RNs. The computations for turnover rate use the number of RNs who left, voluntarily or involuntarily, in the last 12 months, divided by number of total RNs employed, and will be completed in the same way that the figure for the CNAs was computed. The difference is that these figures will be assigned a different point value according to this benchmark because, once again, it is more difficult to hire and train RNs.

Overall: Number of RNs who left, voluntarily or involuntarily, in the past 12 months divided by number of total RNs employed = turnover rate.

Your home's figure _____

Point values are then assigned as follows:

0–12% (5 points)
13–25% (4 points)
26–38% (3 points)
39–51% (2 points)
52–65% (1 point)
66% and above (0 points)

Turnover Rate for Directors of Nursing

> Benchmark: The turnover rate of directors of nursing is less than one over the last year.

The turnover rates for directors of nursing and administrators are calculated differently because these two positions handle more responsibility and tend not to move as frequently as other staff within the home setting.

_____ Number of directors of nursing in the last 12 months

1 (5 points)
2 (3 points)
3 (0 points)

Turnover Rate for Administrators

> Benchmark: The turnover rate of administrators is less than one over the last year.

_____ Number of administrators in the last 12 months

1 (5 points)
2 (3 points)
3 (0 points)

Staff Coverage

Staff coverage outcomes include calculations based on the following criteria:

Percentage of CNA shifts covered by agency staff over the last month

Total number of CNA shifts in a 24-hour period (all shifts, regardless of the number of hours in a shift)

Percentage of nurse shifts covered by agency staff over the last month

Census Rates

Current Occupancy Rate

> Benchmark: Current occupancy rate is above 86%.

The current occupancy rate is computed by dividing the total number of beds by the number of residents. Occupancy rates can be computed by the day, the week, the month, or year, depending upon how you or your facility wants to use the numbers. In some cases, it may be helpful to chart out the occupancy rate on a graph to showcase the trends within your particular facility.

SUMMARY

This chapter addressed the importance of staff employment consistency and availability to residents and the pertinent ACCT benchmarks. The chapter began with a review of the importance of facility outcomes and the relationship of these outcomes to residents' functioning and adaptation. Throughout the chapter, benchmarks to be met in an effort to meet a culture change paradigm within long-term care settings were reviewed, and strategies to address these benchmarks were presented.

DISCUSSION/REFLECTION QUESTIONS

1. Identify benchmark areas within this chapter that you would not have thought of in an effort to create facility outcomes to be more in line with a culture change paradigm.
2. Identify benchmarks within the outcomes domain that you feel have been met within facilities that you either worked in or have been exposed to. Explain why you feel these benchmarks were met.
3. Can you identify three strategies that you and your team could use to address at least one (or up to three) specific benchmarks in the outcomes domain?
4. Think about a service learning project you and your classmates or colleagues could get involved in to help a local facility (or the facility in which you currently work) to help meet one of the benchmarks in the outcomes domain. What steps will you need to put into place to accomplish this goal?

REFERENCES

Arling, G., Kane, R. L., Meuller, C., Bershadsky, J., & Degenholtz, H. B. (2007). Nursing effort and quality of care in nursing home residents. *The Gerontologist, 47*, 672–682.

Castle, N. G., & Engberg, J. (2007). The influence of staffing characteristics on quality of care in nursing homes. *Health Services Research, 42*, 1822–1847.

Munn, J. C., & Zimmerman, S. (2006). A good death for residents of long-term care: Family members speak. *Journal of Social Work in End-of-Life & Palliative Care, 2*(3), 45–59.

Sales, A. E., Bostrom, A., Bucknall, T., Draper, K., Fraser, K., Schalm, C., & Warren, S. (2012). The use of data for process and quality improvement in long term care and home care: A systematic review of the literature. *Journal of the American Medical Directors Association, 13*, 102–113.

Schoeneman, K., & Bowman, C. (2006). *Development of the Artifacts of Culture Change Tool: Report of Contract HHSM-500-2005-00076P* (Technical report). Baltimore, MD: Centers for Medicaid & Medicare Services. Retrieved from http://www.artifactsofculturechange.org/Data/Documents/artifacts.pdf

Spilsbury, K., Hewitt, C., Stirk, L., & Bowman, C. (2011). The relationship between nurse staffing and quality of care in nursing care in nursing homes: A systematic review. *International Journal of Nursing Studies, 48*, 732–750.

III

Tools and Resources to Facilitate the Change Process

The chapters in this third and final part of the book provide specific tools and strategies that are essential to the change process to meet the benchmarks outlined in Part II. Each chapter in this section provides some specific examples of how the skills were used to meet the many challenges in the culture change process. The section concludes with a vision for the future.

11

The Assessment Process: Identifying a Road Map for Success

The process of assessment can be a strategy to help facilitate change within any organization. Various streams of thought currently exist regarding the role of assessment and how it can facilitate organizational change. The results of an assessment can provide a snapshot of an organization's current functioning. The specific areas to be worked on can be identified as "benchmarks." The assessment process can also help an organization build a road map for development, or be helpful in identifying goals to be established for a strategic plan. This chapter addresses specific purposes for which the assessment process can be used and identifies strategies to help long-term care facilities develop an assessment process.

ASSESSMENT AS A TOOL FOR SUCCESS

The concept of assessment is widely used to help define "bragging points" within a specific organization or program. Some people fear the assessment process because it can reveal faults within the current milieu of practice in a long-term care setting or agency. This fear often prevents administrators from engaging in specific assessment strategies. Reframing the importance of assessment can help establish it as a process to facilitate success rather than a means of showcasing an agency's deficits. The assessment process can also be used to answer a variety of questions that help guide facility administrators to better understand their services and the impact of those services for their consumers or residents.

The Artifacts of Culture Change Tool (ACCT; Schoeneman & Bowman, 2006) can be used to pose a number of questions as a part of the process to engage and develop a successful, person-centered program and facility. These questions are outlined in Figure 11.1; however, this segment of the chapter will delve into them more fully.

The first question that can be addressed in an assessment process using the ACCT is "What is the culture of the program?" If a facility has not used the ACCT, an initial baseline in which all of the domains are assessed will help identify what the long-term care program/facility/home and culture of the care facility and program actually are. This also will help identify the type of care/rehabilitation program available through a given facility and what the culture of the program really is.

The second question to address in an assessment process focuses on the specific components/activities through which care is delivered, and through what dimensions or domains this is done. Each of the domains identified through the ACCT will provide a score or benchmark that

---

- What is the culture of the program?

- What are the components, and how do we fare within each of the domains of the ACCT?

- What changes have been incorporated, into the program/facility since the last assessment period or its inception?

- Why were the changes incorporated, and how?

- What changes are planned for the future? Why?

- What is the plan for changes over the next 6 months, 1 year, or 3 years?

- What is our blueprint for your change process developed through the assessment process?

FIGURE 11.1 Questions That Can Be Considered in the Assessment Process

can be used to help identify where the facility currently is in terms of delivering services in a person-centered way. In addition, the facility staff can use these results to help decide on which activities to embark within specific domains.

Third, staff within a facility can ask what changes have been incorporated into the program/facility since the last assessment period. If a new program is being launched, and the ACCT is being used to help understand the specific dimensions of that program, a benchmark identified on the basis of an initial assessment and then a follow-up will help determine whether and how changes have been made and the extent to which the culture change concept has been implemented. If changes have been made, staff and client interviews may elicit information about how changes were incorporated. This approach will also help the facility identify how to celebrate success and "encourage the heart" (Kouzes & Posner, 2012). Changes made can be documented on a score grid to help build an understanding of progress and/or areas for development. This visual approach to documenting the assessment process can be extremely helpful in showcasing trends over time as well as in establishing short- and long-term plans.

The ACCT can also be helpful in establishing specific benchmarks on which a particular unit would like to work for a designated time period, such as 6 months or a year, or plans can be made for a specific set of benchmarks to be achieved within a 3-year period. Although staff may come and go, a savvy administrator may have a vision for where he or she would like to take the facility/home/program over a 3- to 5-year period. The ACCT can help identify specific benchmarks that can be used to determine these goals and establish a blueprint, which could remain in place despite staff changes.

The success of the ACCT can be facilitated through input from a variety of stakeholders, not merely those in key administrative positions. These stakeholders include staff, consumers/clients, administrators, and directors of key departments. Input can be gathered with the ACCT itself (see Chapter 4 for a lengthier discussion of this instrument) as well as through interviews, program documentation, observations, and focus groups.

WHAT IS AN ASSESSMENT?

An assessment is really a process that focuses on collecting information. In the case of assessments within long-term care facilities, the ACCT is designed to collect information related to six specific domains of care/

practice: the environment, the family, the community, care management, leadership practices, and workplace practices and outcomes. Collecting data within these six domains help improve the overall quality of care within the specific facility. Assessment is highly valued by funders and individuals who are responsible for financial outcomes. It can also be used as a way to demonstrate program effectiveness, as we have seen thus far within this chapter.

Assessment is not useless unless it is conducted poorly. Therefore, assessment is also not an end goal but part of a process. It should not be the only information considered when evaluating programs, and it should not consist solely of indexes of consumer satisfaction. In addition, and as discussed in Chapter 4, the assessment process is scientifically guided. Thus, the assessment process is not strictly a series of individual perspectives or opinions.

Assessment also helps one identify or build effective care plans and services within facilities. Implementing benchmarks through the ACCT tool can help identify the characteristics of effective programs. This in turn will assure that meeting the demands and achieving specific outcomes are a result of the ACCT tool, and the planning process it catalyzes. These specific characteristics will include effective and adequate staffing, stable funding and resources, and a consistent service philosophy. Because the ideal is to work toward a culture of person-centered care and dignity toward residents, it would be helpful to ensure that all key players and staff are functioning within the same philosophical perspective. As noted in Chapter 3, various different philosophical paradigms exist. Within the process of assessment, differing and similar philosophical perspectives will undoubtedly surface. These can help determine which staff members can be ambassadors of the change process and which (who are not practicing from a culture change paradigm) should be relegated to teams on which change will be thrust.

Although assessment may be defined in various ways, ranging from patient assessment to organizational assessment, the point of using the ACCT is to identify the extent to which a facility is on the culture change journey and the extent to which change is still necessary. The Pioneer Network recommends that the ACCT be completed a minimum of twice a year, although they strongly recommend that reporting be quarterly, to be consistent with organizational evaluations and reporting. This quarterly assessment will be helpful in identifying incremental changes. Although assessments of responses can be approximates (e.g., responders do not need to count every adaptive handle), providers are encouraged to provide close approximate estimates to ensure the best possible measurements of longitudinal change (Pioneer Network, 2012).

FROM ASSESSMENT TO NEEDS ASSESSMENT

Thus far this chapter has discussed the use of the ACCT for assessment purposes. However, assessment can be short sighted if there is not an apparent linkage between identifying needs, and linking those identified needs with a process with which one's organization can make some positive changes. Ideally, one would want to move the process from an assessment, or identification of needs, to building a blueprint for action, or building a needs assessment.

Needs assessments are defined as tools for helping in the development of decisions. These decision tools can be used to help allocate resources, plan programs and develop programs, and is based upon the perspective that planning programs can help with the growth, expansion or development of programs or services (McKillip, 1998; Royse, Thyer, & Padgett 2010). Thus, the use of data from the ACCT, can be used to help a facility, an administrator or a unit team make decisions about what priorities to set when attempting to move along the culture change journey. The use of the ACCT data can also be helpful in the development of initiatives or programming within a unit or facility. Regardless of how the data is used though, we can develop these strategies through the lens of a needs assessment.

Royse, Thyer, and Padgett (2010) outline four specific types of need which can be components of a needs assessment. These include normative needs, felt needs, expressed needs, and comparative needs. Normative needs include needs that have been defined by an expert. In the case of culture change, experts such as Schoeneman and Bowman (2006) have already identified the normative needs through the ACCT tool, and through the articulation of specific domains for activity or culture change strategies.

The felt needs are needs which tend to be expressed by the consumers. Consumers, for example, may have articulated the need to stay up late and get up in the morning later in the day. They may have also indicated to staff that they would like a wider variety of foods planned into their menus. Each of these thus, would be felt needs or needs expressed by the consumer. If a facility chooses to identify needs or priorities, based upon areas not currently addressed within the ACCT, one could argue that these are felt needs.

Expressed needs, or demand for services, are based upon the voice of consumers who are seeking specific services. This approach is not always the best way to gauge how to build or revise your facility's priorities for change, especially since some of these expressed needs may be biased, or limited to those who would tend to speak up or present their needs. Unfortunately, when planning takes place as a result of expressed needs, quieter or less articulate individuals do not get their specific needs necessarily met. Expressed needs, or needs identified by families or individuals can be used to help identify priorities, but should not be used solely to guide any needs assessment process. As outlined earlier in this book, input from family members is important and critical in any culture change journey, however, we must also ensure that all voices are heard, and not a few outgoing or capable. When used in concert with the areas for growth, identified within the ACCT, expressed needs can help identify which areas to tackle as priorities.

Comparative needs refer to the process of using the needs identified in one facility or area, and inferring these same needs onto either the general population or sister settings (Royse, Thyer & Padgett, 2010). This approach does not always assure that inferring needs from one area to another assures an adequate understanding of the needs. If some needs were identified in one facility (i.e., a dementia care unit), these same needs may not be what the needs were in a sister facility that provided rehabilitation care or assisted living. If a specific long-term care campus offers a continuum of care, it is not realistic to infer that the needs or priorities of one area of care would be the same as other units within the same campus. Hence, it is important to look at assessment data from each specific unit of care (i.e., dementia care, skilled care, etc.) and identify needs per unit, and then as a whole campus, once unit needs are aggregated.

The process on needs assessment, which builds upon data collected in the assessment process, requires careful crafting and input from a variety of stakeholders. Assuring that input from a variety of stakeholders is essential and assuring involvement is also an important dimension. Bargmann (2011) offers some tips for success in the following text box (see Figure 11.2). Needs assessment integrate both evidence about needs (which will be identified through the ACCT) and needs identified by stakeholders and experts who have a vested interest in the change process. Ultimately, the end result of one's assessment and needs assessment process will help identify a road map for action, and hopefully the pathway toward success!

> **TIPS FOR HIGH INVOLVEMENT (BY PEGGY BARGMANN, RN, BSN, CULTURE CHANGE EXPERT)**
>
> Start by gathering the Culture Change Leadership Team. This team should consist of the administrator, the director of nursing, and representatives from each department in the organization. In order to have complete representation of the home, it is important that there be representatives from all levels of the organization. Be sure to include direct care staff members, and at least one family member and one resident. The team is usually [composed] of 15 to 20 people.
>
> Once the team is gathered, have them divide up into groups of three or four and ask each group to complete the [ACCT], ensuring that everyone has input. Once all the groups have completed the tool, a facilitator can bring the large group back together and start down through the tool, enlisting input from all groups to form a final consensus score. For some questions, there will be common agreement on the score. For other questions, there will be a wide variance and the resulting discussion will be lively. By listening, there is much that can be learned during these discussions. The facilitator will need to be sure that all voices in the room have equal input—be sure to be listening to the input from direct care staff, residents, and families. As an example, Question No. 11 states, "Residents can get a bath/shower as often as they would like." The staff may feel that all residents have choice in their bathing times, until a resident informs them that when she moved in she was told what days she was "scheduled" for her shower and didn't realize that she could ask for other days. This could lead to a discussion of how residents are informed and how choice is encouraged and what impact that has on the day-to-day operations.
>
> The process for completing the tool and facilitating the robust discussion can take up to 3 hours. It is a great way for the Culture Change Leadership Team to assess where the home is on its culture change journey, celebrate their accomplishments, and, as a result of the group discussion, generate goals and action plans for their culture change journey. The team can decide how often they want to repeat this process (e.g., every 6 months or annually) in order to assess their progress, celebrate their successes, and revise their goals and action plans, as necessary, to continue on their culture change journey.

FIGURE 11.2 Strategies for High Involvement of Stakeholders

SUMMARY

This chapter begins to address the importance of assessment and to help readers make the connection among assessment, use of the ACCT, and the process of building a database and process to evaluate the impact of culture change efforts. It sets the stage for the process of implementing the use of the ACCT into the actual assessment process.

DISCUSSION/REFLECTION QUESTIONS

1. What strategies could be used to build stakeholder support inside and outside the facility to pursue success?
2. How can the assessment process be used to facilitate a blueprint within your facility or a facility/home where you have worked?
3. What is a needs assessment?
4. How can you engage your group/team within the facility/unit/home where you work in the needs assessment process? How can the ACCT be used as part of a needs assessment process?
5. Working in a group of three to four people, select at least one domain on the ACCT. Using this domain, create a mock assessment (or a real assessment within a facility/home known to the group). Once the assessment has been completed, identify benchmarks that have been accomplished and benchmarks that still need to be reached. Once this step has been completed, identify a plan or blueprint to accomplish benchmarks over a 3-year period.

REFERENCES

Bargman, P., (2011). *Culture Change: Strategies for Success*. A presentation at the National Pioneer Network Culture Change conference, St. Charles, MO.

Kouzes, J., & Posner, B. (2012). *The leadership challenge: How to get extraordinary things done in organizations*. San Francisco, CA: Wiley.

McKillip, J. (1998). Needs analysis: Process and techniques. In L. Bickman & D. Rog (Eds.), *Handbook of applied social research methods*. Thousand Oaks, CA. Sage.

Pioneer Network. (2012). *Assessment tool techniques*. Chicago, IL: Author.

Royse, D., Thyer, B., & Padgett, D. (2010). *Program Evaluation: An introduction*. (5th edition). Belmont,CA: Wadsworth, Cengage Learning.

Schoeneman, K., & Bowman, C. (2006). *Development of the artifacts of culture change tool: report of contract HHSM-500-2005-00076P* (Technical report). Baltimore, MD: Centers for Medicaid & Medicare Services. Retrieved from http://www.artifactsofculturechange.org/Data/Documents/artifacts.pdf

12

From Assessment to Action: Building on the Planning Process

The process of change in long-term care is never an easy one, because systems of care and practice are often engrained and institutionalized. The status quo is always easier than making radical, sweeping changes in any situation. The process of shifting one's thinking paradigms may come more easily to some people than others, and will probably be less painful for younger workers compared to workers who have been on the job for many years. This chapter discusses the process of moving from assessment into active engagement of new practices that were defined in the assessment process. The first step in this process is to understand the stages of change and stages in the transformation process.

A BRIEF GLIMPSE INTO STAGES OF BEHAVIORAL CHANGE

Most people do not willingly embark on a change process. However, all too often we define success as reaching the end goal or vision rather than as making strides toward the end goal. This, too, can characterize the culture change journey and change process. Facility staff should realize that the culture change process is not an either/or proposition but rather a process of stages to be worked through and that require constant evaluation, as noted in Chapter 11. Working through the change process will require behavioral and philosophical changes on the part of the administrator, directors of nursing and the directors of other affiliated professionals, the nursing staff, and the certified nurse assistants (CNAs). Families and residents will also need affirmation that their quest toward person-centered care and dignity, self-worth, and autonomy are acceptable goals. Changing behaviors in the way business is conducted, and moving from assessment to action, is really no different than modifying health-related behaviors. The same stages identified by health promotion experts Prochaska and DiClemente (1983) in their mission to help people change their smoking behaviors can also be applied to moving from assessment to action within the culture change journey. Prochaska and DiClemente's stages-of-change model encompasses following stages: precontemplation, contemplation, preparation, planning, action, and maintenance/follow-up. Each of these stages is discussed in the following few paragraphs.

During the first stage of precontemplation, efforts are made to raise one's consciousness and awareness of how a situation may be different if change were pursued. Training efforts may target staff to help them become aware of the various elements that can affect the system and to create a vision. Efforts at this stage also may be put toward creating an awareness of the culture change paradigm, how person-centered care can be delivered, and vision of what a facility that embraces a culture change approach to care delivery can look like. Interventions at the precontemplation stage may include visits or field trips to facilities engaged in the culture change approach, training sessions, video clips that showcase specific practice domains within facilities that have engaged in culture change efforts, and testimonials from residents and family living in settings that have embarked on the culture change journey.

Within the second stage, contemplation, staff and residents can begin to think about a change process. What would person-centered practices mean within the current setting? What changes could be made to make the facility/home more person directed and less institutionally oriented? These questions are at the core of the contemplation stage. At this point, the goal is to help people within the system begin to think about how to change practices and behaviors; thus, a change in philosophy is crucial. The contemplation stage may integrate opportunities for discussion among team members, residents, and their families about ways to move along the culture change journey. The contemplation stage may precede an actual assessment using the Artifacts of Culture Change Tool (ACCT; Schoeneman & Bowman, 2006), or it may take place after the assessment process has been completed and focus on areas for change and development. Regardless, at this stage, key stakeholders have identified that change will be necessary and begin the process of contemplating how to facilitate change and transformation.

The third stage in the stages-of-change model has been characterized as the preparation phase. During this phase, the key stakeholders identify the resources needed to ensure that the team can take action. This may include an assessment of resources to identify staffing patterns needed, home modifications to be integrated into the facility to focus on a more homelike environment, and/or a list of priorities to be addressed within specific domains on the ACCT. At this stage, specific activities to help build a successful process can be identified. This stage may also include the development of a timeline and a specific evaluation plan to help meet those benchmarks. The preparation phase can also include a "launch" date and celebration to initiate the plan.

The action stage is the fourth one in Prochaska and DiClemente's (1983) framework. In this phase, an active intervention is put into place to help transform or change the behavior or situation of interest. Specific changes to practices and routines take place. Similarly, within the culture change journey, specific changes to care practices may take place. The change from institutional dining to menus and varied food selections would be an examples of changes to dining patterns. Person-centered care practices with consistent assignments for staff may also be an example of activities engaged in that cultivates the action phase.

In the last stage, maintenance/follow-up, individuals reevaluate the changes that have been made and decide whether they can be sustained, or whether other changes need to be made. This phase is the ideal one in which to use the ACCT to reassess the domains. Ideally, a feedback mechanism, or a strategy to share the findings of the intervention/change in practices should also be in place in an effort to showcase how changes have been or should be implemented.

Although changes in the benchmark scores on the ACCT are one indicator of progress on the culture change journey, movement from one stage to the next using the stages-of-change model is also an indicator of success. As a part of the culture change journey, the leadership team may find it helpful to map out some of the specific activities that were accomplished within each stage in this process and the date those activities took place. This can be used to help remind staff, residents, and families of the progress made and activities undertaken within each step in the process. Figure 12.1 provides an illustration of a mural or map that can be used to remind staff, residents, and families of progress.

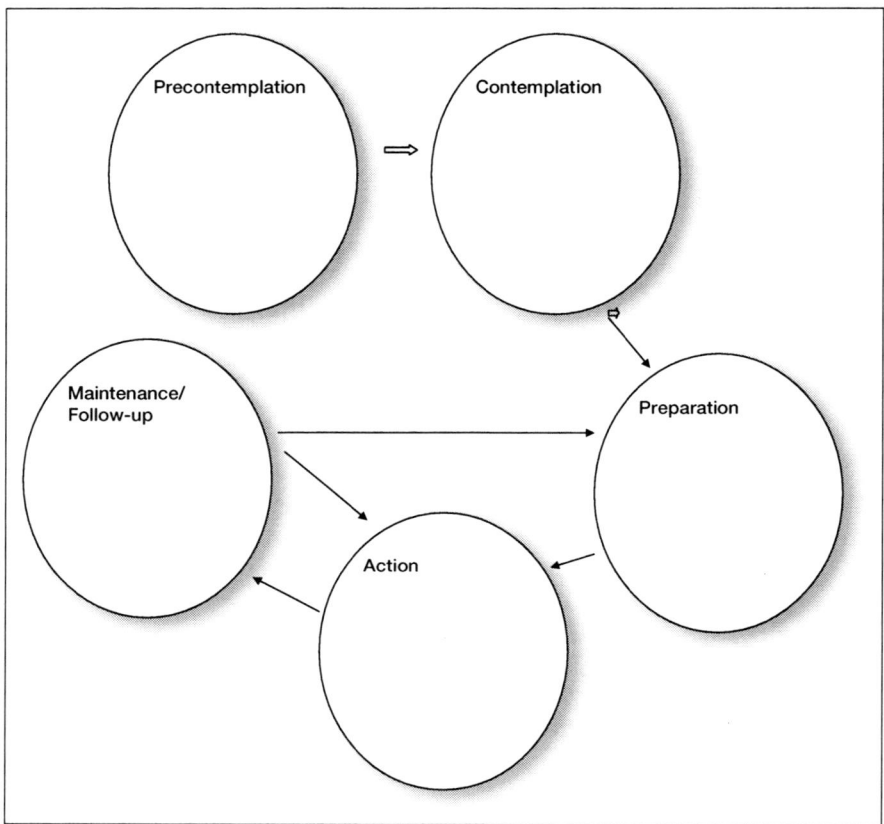

FIGURE 12.1 Road Map for Culture Change Bridging Assessment into Action, Using the Stages-of-Change Framework

Note: To Expand the Use of This Figure in the Form of a Worksheet/Exercise, Within Each of the Circles, Identify What Strategies You Plan to Utilize Within Your Own Culture Change Journey, From Assessment to Action

Stages of Transformation

Some pioneers within the culture change network have identified stages in the process of transformation that facilities have moved through in their quest to become more strongly identifiable as homes that have embarked upon the culture change journey (Action Pact, Inc., n.d.; Lustbader, n.d.; Pioneer Network, n.d.). The first step in this process is to define clear alternatives to the status quo. Individuals should brainstorm a series of clear alternatives to the current practices. For example, the team may want to look at alternative practices to bathing. The first step then would be to brainstorm alternatives to the steps currently in place.

One of the initial steps in the change process is to identify a series of clear alternatives to the current practices. This may need to be done at a meeting with staff and residents, or by a designated culture change team that has been given the task of mobilizing practices and innovations within the ACCT domains. The team may identify, for example, three specific practices that they want to change within a 6-month period. Within a learning circle format, the team may want to brainstorm a series of alternatives (with no idea being ruled out) and then choose specific strategies to mobilize each idea. The staff may want to then vote on the best alternatives to begin to initiate as part of the change process.

The Process of Change

The actual process of change within any setting can be painful. People or organizations gravitate toward the status quo, and change can prove to be difficult and challenging. Superficial changes may act as a bandage of sorts for serious underlying problems in the foundation; thus, it is important to be mindful of the kinds of changes that may necessary and to dialogue about what is at the foundation of changes. Will the changes cover up some long-standing problems, or will they definitely help mobilize all parties toward a different place along the culture change continuum? Although there is no easy answer or any hard and fast rule as to how to assess whether the changes are superficial or deep, the important component in the process is honest, open, and creative dialogue.

Within open and honest dialogue, it is important for all members of the leadership team to agree that no ideas are stupid and are open for evaluation, consideration, and discussion. The leadership team must be prepared to address issues and "practice what they preach." Honest dialogue is a must, and both negativity and enthusiasm should be aired. This approach to honest dialogue will heighten each person's awareness of the situation, the process of change, and the role that benchmarks will play in helping to move the culture change process along. New models of supervision should be included along with the honest dialogue. The next section addresses this approach.

ENCOURAGE NEW MODELS OF SUPERVISION

Supervision practices will play a central role in the movement of a culture change and the shift from the assessment process into the action process. Supervision practices will probably need to move from being task oriented to being relationship driven. Chapter 8 discussed leadership practices at some length on the basis of a framework developed by Kouzes and Posner (1987). Supervision that embraces activities that fall within the realm of five specific leadership practices (challenging the process, modeling the way, inspiring a shared vision, encouraging the heart, and enabling others to act) could form the basis of a new paradigm of supervision. This new approach could easily help staff build upon new strategies for engaging in the care practices of residents/people living within a home/facility.

An initial step in the engagement of a new model for supervision can start with the assessment process, whereby staff/residents and/or the leadership team identify and explore care practices that they would like to include as part of the movement to embrace new benchmarks in the care practice arena. As mentioned earlier in this chapter, dialogue to help facilitate a process for reaching these benchmark items will begin with the development of a learning circle for the discussion of practice care issues. A revised approach to supervision would include the development of ongoing team interaction, as well as dialogue. Accomplishing the tasks will not be as important as encouraging the vision among the team members.

New models of supervision will also help cultivate a team approach and facilitate staff engagement. The end result of this approach will ideally lead to strategies to reduce staff turnover, because a relationship-oriented approach to team building will help build strategies for staff to feel engaged in their work and valued as helping professionals.

HELP THE CARE STAFF AND CNAs TO BE RESPONSIVE

Within the action phase of the culture change implementation process, the care staff and CNAs need to feel empowered and valued. Given that they work on the front lines with the residents, management strategies are needed to help support and value the relationships CNAs have with residents and the work in which these members of the care team are engaged. A strategy that can be helpful in building the responsiveness of care staff and CNAs includes the elimination of middle management layers. The myriad red tape required for decision making and reporting can detract from time spent in relationships with residents.

Consistent assignments for staff and attendants can be extremely helpful in moving the care plan assessment items into action. The consistency of staff working with the same residents helps the residents build trust and ensures that the staff understand and anticipate their needs. In Chapter 9, which addressed care practices, the scientific literature pointed to the importance of consistent staffing when considering quality outcomes and resident satisfaction. The commitment to the process of a consistent assignment also facilitates the movement from assessment to action and a new step along the stages-of-change continuum.

Additional innovative strategies that will engage the responsiveness of care staff includes valuing the observations and relationships that the CNAs have developed with the residents. Too often, care planning and care conferences involve only the professional staff and minimize the input that CNAs can have to contribute to the process. The involvement of the CNAs in these care planning and care conferences can help facilities achieve many of the care practice benchmarks within the care practice domains, because much of CNAs' primary responsibility involves helping support the residents' autonomy and well-being.

The process of supporting responsiveness on the part of the care team ultimately is based on the concept of supporting a team. Supervisory and management practices need to be built upon the concept of the value of each member of the team and the belief that each team member plays an integral role in mobilizing the assessed needs into action. The concept of a team approach to mobilizing any one or all of the practice domains is key in efforts to transform the ACCT benchmarks from an idea (precontemplation/contemplation) to fruition (action), and then institutionalizing these practices into action (maintenance) and evaluating their impact (assessment).

Create a Homelike Environment

The last step in moving from assessment to action includes the ultimate goal: to create a homelike environment. In efforts to reach this goal, and mobilize the assessment process into action, several steps are necessary. First, one must ensure that all staff are cross-trained so they are capable of covering for other staff and of carrying out more than their assigned tasks. The inclusion of family members in the decision-making process moves the process from one that is patronizing to one that is built on partnership and recognition of individuality. This in turn will cultivate a community and help build relationships. The environment practice domain within the ACCT also supports strategies to facilitate the redesigning of traditional, institutional-looking structures to ones that make the surroundings look more homelike and that more accurately reflect the preferences and values shared by the residents.

Last but not least is the importance of building proactive relationships with the surveyors. Surveyors can make or break the success of a culture change journey within a facility. Hence, the importance of cultivating cooperative relationships with them, and ensuring that they will interpret the regulations to support a person-centered approach, will be paramount in a successful transformation in one's home. Chapter 15 addresses regulatory issues and provides some hints for success. However, a supportive relationship, built on respect and communication, ultimately is an essential building block to fostering the implementation of culture change strategies within a facility. Proactive relationships will also help with blurring the lines of the current regulations and providing an interpretation of the guidelines that are more in line with practices within the ACCT.

SUMMARY

This chapter examined the change process and provided a framework to help readers conceptualize the constructs of change. Prochaska and DiClemente's (1983) stages-of-change model was presented, along with examples of how this model can be used to support a culture change paradigm move from the assessment process to action. The chapter concluded with a series of steps that can be helpful in this process.

DISCUSSION/REFLECTION QUESTIONS

1. *Consider the domain your team used in Chapter 11 to conduct an assessment. How would your team examine each of the stages identified in the stages-of-change model to build a blueprint to move from assessment to action?*
2. *What supervision strategies would you recommend to help move the process from assessment to action?*
3. *What roadblock or challenges may prevent you and your team from developing positive and proactive relationships with your surveyor?*

REFERENCES

Action Pact, Inc. (n.d.). *A tale of transformation: Four stages to tell a story* [DVD]. Chicago, IL: The Pioneer Network.
Kouzes, J., & Posner, B. (1987). *The leadership challenge: How to get extraordinary things done in organizations*. San Francisco, CA: Jossey-Bass.

Lustbader, W. (n.d.). *The pioneer challenge: A radical change in the culture of nursing homes*. Rochester, NY: The Pioneer Network.
Pioneer Network, (n.d.) The Culture Change story.
Prochaska, J. O., & DiClemente, C. C. (1983). Stages and processes of self-change of smoking: Toward an integrative model of change. *Journal of Consulting and Child Psychology, 51,* 390–395.
Schoeneman, K., & Bowman, C. (2006). *Development of the artifacts of culture change tool: Report of contract HHSM-500-2005-00076P* (technical report). Baltimore, MD: Centers for Medicaid & Medicare Services. Retrieved from http://www.artifactsofculturechange.org/Data/Documents/artifacts.pdf

13

Partners for Change: Residents and Family

This chapter focuses on families and their involvement in the process of facilitating a paradigm of culture change. If you are a family member with a loved one currently in a long-term care facility and are reading this for the first time, it may almost be too late for you to take advantage of the ideas presented. Family and consumers (residents) both play a vital role in defining the care and environment of the facility they call home. Thus, this chapter is designed to help readers understand how families and individuals who receive care can be partners in the planning and implementation process.

CONSUMER PARTICIPATION—WHAT DO WE KNOW ABOUT THE ROLE?

The disability arena has a long-established trend of consumer participation and its benefits for individuals and their families. However, family and consumer participation within the case management process, or as active partners have only recently become the norm. Within the disability arena, the self-advocacy movement gave rise to the importance of consumer and family participation in the pathway to securing person-centered and enhanced services. Improvements in services within this arena were facilitated by partnerships with family and consumers. In fact, these groups often drove or spearheaded changes within the disability arena (Braddock, 1992; Itzhaky & York, 1991; Jurkowski, 1997; Jurkowski, Jovanovic, & Rowitz, 2002; Keys & Foster-Fishman, 2000; Lord, 1987; Miller & Keys, 1996; Zimmerman & Rappaport, 1988). In fact, research showed that when families and consumers participated as advocates or partners in the service network's governance process, they were at least five times more likely to receive health care and social services than if they had not participated (Jurkowski, 1997). Although this finding is dated, this early study helps us understand why the disability movement and service delivery arena has become partnership driven and how a person-centered approach to service delivery and care has transpired. Similar to the pioneer movement and culture change movement today, consumers two decades ago wanted to move away from being recipients of services to active partners in the planning process (Heller, Peterson, & Miller, 1996), which led to the shift in paradigm within the disability arena.

The concept of *empowerment*, which originated within the mental health arena in regard to psychiatric patients, has also been an important vehicle for change and a direct pathway for people with psychiatric impairments to become active consumer participants. The concept of empowerment actually originates from Soliman (1976), who suggested that true empowerment cultivated by change agents was embraced by five key elements:

1. Collaborative partnerships with clients, client groups, and constituents
2. A focus or emphasis on client strengths, capacities, thoughts, and resources
3. A dual working focus with people and their social and physical environments
4. The assumption that subjects are active participants and claimants
5. The selective channeling of energies to historically disempowered groups and individuals (p. 24).

Andonian and MacRae (2011) explored the importance of older adults and their involvement in fostering social participation. These authors used the photovoice method to examine the role of social participation among older adults in California. Photovoice—the use of photography to showcase social networks and social relationships—revealed that participants valued a sense of belonging and unconditional acceptance. Andonian and MacRae also found that promoting a sense of membership and importance with loved ones helped promote a healthy sense of identity and being. The results of their study point to the importance of staff roles in facilitating connections with others and of continuing to value the relationships with others, including family members.

Over the past decade, attempts have been made to integrate consumer voice into the activities of long-term care facilities, although many of these attempts have been perceived as token rather than substantive. The ombudsman program, federally mandated and delivered in every state, supports resident councils within facilities, as well as family councils. The councils are charged with the task of incorporating residents', consumers', and families' voices into the workings of the facility. Unfortunately, shortcomings in leadership, training, and support often marginalize these councils' impact and effectiveness. Although it is clear that when residents and families are involved in the planning process, a partnership is much more likely, work is still needed to help families and residents become more involved as partners. Some of this work may have to take place prior to entry into long-term care settings, such as advanced planning to address where functional limitations may have an impact. However, strategies to involve the family and resident in sharing their voice during the actual planning of resources within facilities also are necessary. The remainder of this chapter addresses these areas.

ADVANCE PLANNING

All too often, by the time an individual needs long-term care, he or she is not going to be the best advocate of his or her specific needs and preferences. This is not to suggest that they do not have preferences at this point but that they may be incapacitated to the point that they are not able to advocate for their needs. In such cases, family members will be the ones to create a profile of the individual and reflect who and what their loved one represents. For example, consider the case of Martin. Martin had been an accountant for the duration of his career. He was an active community member, served on his local city council, was a Boy Scout leader, a member of the local horticultural society, an avid sports fan, and a golfer. Afflicted by a case of meningitis at age 76, Martin became severely dependent on his family, was forced to give up his driver's license, and needed assistance with his activities of daily living. Although he still was cognitively intact, his mobility was significantly impaired, and he required home health care aides to assist him with bathing, dressing, shaving, and showering. Although he had been an easygoing gentle soul throughout his life, he often was combative with the home health aides because of his own frustration with the situation and his feelings of loss regarding his diminished independence. Assessed as an aggressive person by the home health staff, he was often treated with a level of guardedness by aides, and conversations between the aides and Martin were often limited.

After Martin's passing, his wife received several condolence telephone calls and visits from the men who had served as home health aides during the last several months of Martin's life. They all commented that they wished they had known Martin during his active days, and wished they had been aware of his many networks, outlets, and accomplishments when they had been working with Martin. One aide confessed that had he been aware of Martin's background as a person, that he would have treated Martin in a completely different manner. These visits and comments were a direct result of the aides having the opportunity to read about Martin in his obituary and discovering how multifaceted, accomplished, and talented Martin was.

This example is not unique in the world of elders, people with mobility impairments and disabilities, people who are hospitalized, or people in long-term care settings. All too often, what the care staff sees is an individual with frailties and limitations, rather than gifts and talents. Unfortunately, admissions to long-term care settings and homes often revolve around some form of medical crisis, so the admission process also often minimizes the process of getting to know the person and instead focuses on getting to know his or her needs (i.e., the medical model paradigm). Consequently, it would be very useful for individuals and families to prepare in advance a "Personal Preference Inventory Plan" or PPI, which can serve as a background to the individual and help facilitate the care team's understanding of the person and facilitate person-centered care.

BUILDING A PERSONAL PREFERENCE INVENTORY

The PPI was designed to be a tool for helping staff in a hospital or care facility better know who the patient/resident is and to make support workers aware of the personality attributes and preferences that the individual has. It also shares information that help care staff better understand the individual's personal history, culture, values, preferences, and, in some cases, philosophies about one's lifestyle, which will help them understand the person. The PPI ideally should be developed long before one is in need of long-term care, but in the worst case scenario it can be completed by family members in the event the individual is incapacitated in some way. If the person has suffered a stroke or has dementia, and all facets of memory are not working optimally, the PPI, if completed by family members, can greatly assist in building an understanding of who the individual is.

Once completed, a copy of the PPI materials can be left at the front door of the resident's room, preferably in a mailbox. The benefits of this approach would be that a new aide or employee would have an opportunity to get to know something about the person prior to working with him or her, and the material is easily accessible. The same would hold true for volunteers, who may not necessarily have access to medical or file information. The PPI also helps bridge a person's lifetime preferences and accomplishments with the current day and practice of care. People who are partially or fully incapacitated may have difficulty easily communicating who they are and what their preferences are. Another option for storing this information would be on a stick drive or on a computer monitor that is available for patient information, outside resident rooms.

Each of the PPI's seven domains are designed to help capture the major values and experiences that a person may have been involved with, experienced, or valued over the course of his or her lifetime. These domains include social supports and family (family/social support domain), areas of one's previous work and training (vocational/occupational domain), extracurricular activities (recreational domain), education/academic history (intellectual domain), one's spirituality/religion (spirituality domain), physical history and condition (physical/well-being domain), and one's mental health history (mental vitality domain). The next section of this chapter articulates the components of the PPI.

COMPONENTS OF A PERSONAL PREFERENCE INVENTORY

When building a PPI, it is important to understand the specific components and be able to address these components when building a plan. In this section, each of the seven domains of the PPI are explained, a worksheet is presented, and a sample of a completed worksheet is provided to help illustrate the specific components of the plan.

When developing one's PPI, it is helpful if the responses to the questions are written in a person-first language (i.e., "I …"). This approach helps personalize the inventory and enliven the person and his or her attributes.

Family/Social Support

The family/social support domain is designed to help showcase family members, friends, and other members of one's social support system. All too often, relatives and friends who live afar and are not able to travel frequently will not be included in this domain. Also, individuals with dementia may talk about a loved one or friend, but the care team may have no idea who the person is or why he or she is a part of the resident's life. The questions in this domain are designed to help build a profile of the resident's family and social life. Each subarea identified within the domain encompasses a variety of questions to help build a profile within the subcategories. These subcategories include marriage/partnership, children/grandchildren, and social supports.

Marriage/Partnership

Marriage or long-term relationships are generally an aspect of one's social network. Within this subcategory, the questions help others understand the courtship, romance, and relationship one has with his or her spouse. Questions to help convey the uniqueness of this relationship include the following:

Are you married currently, and who is your spouse?

What is your spouse's name and age (approximate) or year of birth?

How long have you been in this relationship, and how long have you been married?

What stories can you share about your courtship and how you met?

Have you had previous marriages/relationships that have been significant in your life?

Describe these people, and describe how you met, or share something about your relationship.

Has abuse (physical, mental, or financial) been a part of this relationship or any relationships with significant partners?

Children/Grandchildren

Do you have children? If so, how many, and what is/are their gender? Are there any specific things about your children that you are proud of (academic achievements, careers/jobs, areas of interest, etc.)? What are their names/birthdates? Where do they live?

Do you have grandchildren? Who are they, what are their names and years of birth, and do they have any special accomplishments?

Are there any interests or activities that you are especially proud of or involved in with either your children or grandchildren?

Are there any special activities that you would like to reminisce about with your children or grandchildren?

Siblings

Do you have siblings and, if so, what is their gender and age difference to you? What was your relationship like with your siblings?

Social Supports

Are there any special friends, long term or short term, who are important to you in your life?

How did you become friends, and/or how has your relationship developed over time?

What are some of the specific activities you enjoy doing with these special people in your life?

In summary, this domain helps the care staff understand a resident's social support network. It also provides an overview of the people and range of people involved in a person's life and the quality of those relationships.

Vocational/Occupational Domain

The way one earns a living or contributes to his or her family income plays a role in defining one's being. The questions for this domain elicit information about one's history within his or her work or occupational fields across his or her lifetime. Sometimes knowing a person's profession does not allow complete understanding of a resident's behaviors or mannerisms, but understanding some of the specific roles that the individual had undertaken in the past may help care staff understand agitation or behavior. This domain includes work history, roles held, and training or special recognition.

Work History

What are some of the places where you have worked? What city were the jobs in, and for what length of time did you work?

Are there any jobs that were more enjoyable or significant than others?

Roles Held

What roles have you held within specific jobs? Have you been promoted over time and, if so, in what capacity?

What jobs did you enjoy the most?

What jobs or roles did you enjoy the least?

What jobs or roles are you most proud of?

Have there been any significant accomplishments that you want to brag about?

Military History

Do you have a military history?

What branch of service did you serve in?

What era of combat were you in?

What military honors do you hold?

Training and Special Recognition

Are there any specific training courses that you have participated in that were of importance to you?

Are there any recognitions or awards that were important to you or that you were proud of?

Recreational Domain

Hobbies

What hobbies have been important in your life?

Are there some hobbies that you would have liked to have participated in, but have not?

Are there some hobbies that you would not like to be a part of, and why?

Have you been a collector of any sorts and, if so, of what?

Special Talents

Are there any special talents that you have developed over the course of your lifetime that have been significant?

Are there any leadership roles you have played in building these talents for others in the community?

Artistic Interests

What are your specific artistic interests (e.g., theater, opera, sculpting, painting, singing, music, etc.)?

Describe your favorite (or as many as you'd like to share) areas within the arts.

Sporting Interests

What are your specific sporting interests?

What sports have you played recreationally or professionally over your lifetime?

What sports do you enjoy watching now?

Travel

Where have you traveled over the course of your lifetime if travel has been an interest for you?

What do you enjoy about travel?

What have been some of your favorite places to travel, and are there some specific aspects of the culture that you would like to retain?

What ethnic foods do you enjoy?

Are there some ethnic foods that you do not like?

Movie Interests

What types of movies do you enjoy watching?

Who are some of your favorite actors and actresses?

What are some of your favorite movies?

What are some movies that you do not like?

Authors of Interest

If you are a reader, which authors are you especially interested in reading?

Have you used books on CD or books on tape?

Have you ever used an e-reader or tablet?

What types of books are you interested in reading?

Games of Interest

What types of games have you been interested in playing over your lifetime?

Are there board games or video games that you enjoy and, if so, what are they?

Computer Literacy

Are you able to use a computer?

Do you have an e-mail address?

Do you use a webcam to visit with your loved ones?

Have you used Internet search engines to find information about subjects you are interested in?

Organizational Affiliation

Over the course of your life, what specific organizations have you been a member of?

Which of these organizations have you been involved with for a long period of time, or have received lifetime recognition for? (These can include service-related organizations, e.g., the Knights of Columbus, Kiwanis, Rotary Club, Masons, etc.)

Civic Engagement

What community organizations or community leadership roles have you held during your lifetime? These can include elected roles (mayor, city or county boards), appointed roles (chairperson for a fundraiser or parent–teacher association) and service-related organizations.

Intellectual Domain

The areas that challenge one's intellectual capacity are also of interest and may require support and recognition in one's later years. These items include one's education, training, and other accomplishments

Education

What was the highest level of education you earned?

What are your academic or educational achievements?

Training

What special training courses have you been involved with over your lifetime?

Academic Accomplishments

What honors or awards have you received that you have been proud of during your lifetime?

Languages

What languages do you speak?

What languages do you write?

What languages can you read?

Spirituality Domain

Religious Background/History

Over the course of your lifetime, describe some of your background or history with religion or faith/spirituality.

Spiritual Practices

What are some of your specific spiritual practices (e.g., if Catholic, do you pray the Rosary; if Muslim, do you pray several times per day; if Jewish, how important are weekly Shabbat meals?)

What practices would you like to maintain as you age that have been an important part of your lifestyle?

Favorite Religious Celebrations or Holidays

What are some of your favorite religious celebrations or holidays? Describe your memories of these celebrations and/or how you would like to celebrate.

What Are Some Treasured Memories About Your Spiritual/Religious Background?

What traditions have been in your family related to your spirituality?

What are some of your favorite memories of celebrations?

Physical/Well-Being Domain

Physical Health and Values About Staying Healthy

What are some of your values about maintaining your physical health and mobility?

What have been some of your health routines over the course of your lifetime, and most recently?

Do you have any specific food or dietary practices that are part of your well-being (i.e., vegan, vegetarian, soy products, etc.)?

Mental Vitality Domain

Mental Vitality and Values About Mental Vitality

What are some of your values about maintaining your mental health and vitality?

What have some of your health routines been over the course of your lifetime, and most recently, to maintain your mental vitality?

Do you have any specific food or dietary practices that are part of your well-being (e.g., vegan, vegetarian, soy products, etc.) to promote your mental vitality?

Health History

What is significant in your health history that you want to share over and above what has been recorded in your health records?

Is there any other significant information not found in the health record that needs to be shared? If so, what would it be?

Family members and the resident may also want to include in the PPI any specific terms or words used to describe events or situations. This may also include specific terminology or names that the resident would like to be called. Table 13.1 provides an overview of the instrument, with potential questions. Table 13.2 provides the same overview, except the individual in the case study, Martin, is described on the PPI.

TABLE 13.1 Personal Preference Inventory Guide

Domain	Key Questions to Elicit Information About the Individual
Family/ social support	*Marriage/partnership:* Are you married currently, and who is your spouse? What is his or her name and age (approximate) or year of birth? How long have you been in this relationship, and how long have you been married? What stories can you share about your courtship and how you met?
	Have you had previous marriages/relationships that have been significant in your life? Describe these people, and describe how you met, or share something about your relationship.
	Children/grandchildren: Do you have children? If so, how many, and what are their gender? Are there any specific things about your children that you are proud of (academic achievements, careers/jobs, areas of interest, etc.)? What are their names/birthdates, and so on? Where do they live?
	Do you have grandchildren? What are their names, years of birth, and any special accomplishments?
	Are there any interests or activities that you are especially proud of or involved in with either your children or grandchildren?
	Are there any special activities that you would like to reminisce about with your children or grandchildren?
	Siblings: Do you have siblings and, if so, what is their gender and age difference to you?
	What was your relationship like with your siblings?
	Social Supports: Are there any special friends, long term or short term, who are important to you in your life?
	How did you become friends and/or how has your relationship developed over time?
	What are some of the specific activities that you enjoy doing with these special people in your life?
Vocational/ occupational	*Work history:* What are some of the places you have worked? What cities have you worked in, and for what length of time?
	Are there any jobs that were more enjoyable or significant than others?

Domain	Key Questions to Elicit Information About the Individual
	Roles held: What roles have you held within specific jobs? Have you been promoted over time, and in what capacity? What jobs did you enjoy the most? What jobs or roles did you enjoy the least? What jobs or roles are you most proud of? Have there been any significant accomplishments that you want to brag about? *Military history:* Do you have a military history? What branch of service did you serve in? What era of combat were you in? What military honors do you hold? *Training and special recognition:* Are there any specific training courses you have participated in that were important to you? Are there any recognitions or awards that were important to you or that you were proud of?
Recreational	*Hobbies:* What hobbies have been important in your life? Are there some hobbies that you would have liked to have participated in, but have not? Are there some hobbies that you would not like to be a part of and why? Have you been a collector of any sorts, and if so, of what? *Special talents:* Are there any special talents that you have developed over the course of your lifetime that have been significant? Are there any leadership roles you have played in building these talents for others in the community? *Artistic interests:* What are your specific artistic interests (e.g., theater, opera, sculpting, painting, singing, music, etc.)? Describe what your favorites are in any (or as many) areas within the arts. *Sporting interests:* What are your specific sporting interests? What sports have you played recreationally or professionally over your lifetime? What sports do you enjoy watching now? *Travel:* Where have you traveled over the course of your lifetime if travel has been an interest for you? What do you enjoy about travel?

(continued)

TABLE 13.1 Personal Preference Inventory Guide (*continued*)

Domain	Key Questions to Elicit Information About the Individual
	What have been some of your favorite places to travel, and are there some specific aspects of the culture that you would like to retain?
	What ethnic foods do you enjoy?
	Are there some ethnic foods that you do not like?
	Movie interests: What types of movies do you enjoy watching?
	Who are some of your favorite actors and actresses?
	What are some of your favorite movies?
	What are some movies that you do not like?
	Authors of interest: If you are a reader, which authors are you especially interested in reading?
	Have you used books on CD or books on tape?
	Have you ever used an e-reader or tablet??
	What types of books are you interested in reading?
	Games of interest: What types of games have you been interested in playing over your lifetime?
	Are there board games, or video games, that you enjoy? If so, what are they?
	Computer literacy: Are you able to use a computer?
	Do you have an e-mail address?
	Do you use a webcam to visit with your loved ones?
	Have you used Internet search engines to find information about subjects you are interested in?
	Organizational affiliation: Over the course of your life, what specific organizations have you been a member of?
	Which of these organizations have you been involved with for a long period of time, or have received lifetime recognition for? (These can include service-related organizations, e.g., the Knights of Columbus, Kiwanis, Rotary Club, Masons, etc.)
	Civic engagement: What community organizations or community leadership roles have you held during your lifetime? These can include elected roles (mayor, city or county boards), appointed roles (chairperson for a fundraiser or parent–teacher association) and service-related positions.
Intellectual	*Education:* What was the highest level of education you earned?
	What are your academic or educational achievements?
	Training: What special training courses have you been involved with over your lifetime?

Domain	Key Questions to Elicit Information About the Individual
	Academic accomplishments: What honors or awards have you received that you have been proud of during your lifetime? *Languages:* What languages do you speak? What languages do you write? What languages can you read?
Spirituality	*Religious background/history:* Over the course of your lifetime, describe some of your background or history with religion or faith/spirituality. *Spiritual practices:* What are some of your specific spiritual practices (e.g., if Catholic, do you pray the Rosary; if Muslim, do you pray several times per day; if Jewish, how important are weekly Shabbat meals?)? What practices would you like to maintain as you age that have been an important part of your lifestyle? *Favorite religious celebrations or holidays:* What are some of your favorite religious celebrations or holidays? Describe your memories of these celebrations and/or how you would like to celebrate. *What are some treasured memories about your spiritual/religious background?* What traditions have been in your family related to your spirituality? What are some of your favorite memories of celebrations?
Physical/ well-being	*Physical health and values about staying healthy:* What are some of your values about maintaining your physical health and mobility? What have some of your health routines been over the course of your lifetime, and most recently? Do you have any specific food or dietary practices that are part of your well-being (i.e., vegan, vegetarian, soy products, etc.)?
Mental vitality	*Mental vitality and values about mental vitality:* What are some of your values about maintaining your mental health and vitality? What have some of your health routines been over the course of your lifetime, and most recently, to maintain your mental vitality? Do you have any specific food or dietary practices that are part of your well-being (e.g., vegan, vegetarian, soy products, etc.) to promote your mental vitality? *Health history:* What is significant in your health history that you want to share over and above what has been recorded in your health records? Is there any other significant information not found in the health record that needs to be shared? If so, what would it be?

TABLE 13.2 Sample Personal Preference Inventory for "Martin"

Domain	Martin's Responses to Key Questions
Family/ social support	*Marriage/partnership:* I have been married for 49 years and my wife's name is Lori. She is 10 years younger than I. We met while visiting a mutual friend in the hospital, about 4 years before we began our courtship. We were reunited with each other at a local church when Lori was singing in the church choir, and I was visiting my brother and sister-in-law. Our first date was to a wrestling match, and we have laughed over the date for years to follow. Lori forgot her eyeglasses at home, and could not see any of the wrestling match! Over the years of our marriage, Lori has kept me happy and content with her domestic talents. She has always enjoyed working in the kitchen and preparing lovely baked goods. We have always enjoyed special occasions and the holidays—especially Christmas, Easter, and Thanksgiving. Lori always liked to decorate our home for the holidays. I am the fourth born of eight children and have been especially close to my next brother Fred, who was born 10 months after me. The two of us spent the most time together. My youngest two sisters are also close to me, because I married late in life, and growing up, they took part in many activities with me. *Children/grandchildren:* I have raised four children, three boys and a girl. My sons currently are 56, 46, and 42 years of age, and my daughter is 54 years old. All of my children are college educated, and two of my children have earned their PhDs, one in music and one in business. My youngest son works as a consultant with his MBA, and my daughter is a social worker. I am very proud of their academic achievements. My children live in various parts of the world—two live in Europe, and two live nearby in Colorado. My eldest son, Martin, lives in Austria and works for the European Music Academy as director. My second son is working in London for the Huffington Investment Group. My daughter and youngest son live nearby in Denver suburbs. Currently, I have six grandchildren, ranging in age from 4 to 27. The oldest two grandchildren, Stephan and Jami, both have two sons, who are my great grandchildren. My other grandchildren, Rosemarie (22), Baker (18), Douglas (9), and Wayne (4), also bring me great joy. The youngest four children live in Castlerock and Aurora, CO, and all have participated in gifted education programs. The youngest two boys are expert skiers, while Rosemarie is currently studying at Stanford University in a neuroscience master's/PhD program. All the grandchildren have earned at least one postsecondary degree and are very hard working. My oldest grandson, Stephan, is working within the international trade arena, while Jami is a sculptor/photographer. During the growing years, all grandchildren would spend a week at a time during the summer months with their grandmother and me at our cabin in Cape Cod. *Social supports:* My wife and I have been very involved in our church community over the course of our marriage.

Domain	Martin's Responses to Key Questions
	We have developed a large network of friends, through our activity in the church choir, and have kept many of these friends throughout our lifetime.
	Some of the specific activities that we have been active. over the course of our lifetime have included bowling, our church/faith-based community, scouting, gardening (Local Horticultural Society), the Knights of Columbus, and the Kiwanis Club. I also enjoyed model railroading and was voted most creative model railroader at a national convention.
	During my retirement years, I sat on the local city council and chaired the budget/revenue committee.
	Each of these specific activities has led me to develop unique relationships and friendships with others.
Vocational/ occupational	*Work history:* I worked for 42 years at the Colorado Telephone System, when it was a public entity, and I retired in 1986.
	By the time I ended my career, I served as the Vice President for Methods Development, a role which I held for the last 5 years of my career,
	Roles held: I began my career with the Colorado Telephone Company as a mail boy, delivering mail to people throughout the organization. I was well liked, outgoing, humorous, and witty (unfortunately, my stroke has affected my speech now). Most people throughout the organization knew me and, in time, I found myself in demand for various jobs, simply because of my reputation. I progressed and worked in the methods accounting division, and eventually was promoted to Chief for Methods Accounting. Once in this role, I progressively worked myself toward the Vice President of Methods Development. I enjoyed each and every job, so I cannot say there was one role I enjoyed more than others. The accomplishments that I am most proud of include the automation of our billing department, which pushed our entire billing division to become automated rather than manual. I was also pleased with several of the new initiatives that we implemented to streamline the billing process.
	Training and special recognition: My initial training was in accounting at a local junior college. Through a variety of night and weekend classes, I was able to eventually complete my MBA, a degree I was very proud to receive. I also have an engineering degree.
	Through my work and career, I was able to earn numerous patents for my work. In fact, I have received over 25 patents!
	I was acknowledged as one of the most innovative within my field and given a lifetime achievement award through the Telephone Pioneers of America, just after my retirement in 1985.
Recreational	*Hobbies:* Hobbies that I have enjoyed throughout my life include stamp collecting, gardening, Boy Scouts (I attained the highest rank, Eagle Scout), collecting coupons, and music.
	The hobbies most important to me include gardening, singing, improvisation comedy, and mentoring young men through Boy Scouts.

(continued)

TABLE 13.2 Sample Personal Preference Inventory for "Martin" (continued)

Domain	Martin's Responses to Key Questions
	Over my lifetime, I would have liked to have been able to spend more time watching old movies.
	Stamp collecting is the hobby that I most enjoy, having been exposed to it as a child through my father.
	Special talents:
	Some specific talents that I have include team building and staff negotiations. I am particularly proud of these skills.
	Some of the leadership roles that I have undertaken within the community include member of the city council and member of various planning committees. I was also the chairperson for the methods development group within the city council of Pinecrest Community, CO, a role I maintained the longest tenure—9 years.
	Artistic interests:
	My wife and I enjoy the arts. We have had season tickets for the Denver Symphony Orchestra for at least 25 years. We also enjoy opera.
	Two of my favorite musicians are Benny Goodman and Tony Bennett. Although we have seen them perform live numerous times, each seems like the first! I can never get enough from dear old Joli! (Al Jolson).
	Sporting interests:
	My sporting interests include golf, baseball, football, curling, bowling, and hockey.
	I played golf professionally in my early to late 20s but have also played on community league amateur baseball and hockey teams for "old timers" following my retirement.
	I still enjoy watching hockey, football, curling, and the Olympics.
	Travel:
	Travel has been a keen interest for my wife and I. We have traveled extensively throughout my retirement, and have visited all modern Wonders of the World, six continents, and the Arctic Circle.
	We have most enjoyed traveling through southeast Asia and the Slavic countries in Europe.
	I would like to retain some of my Slavic heritage. Notice that I have a Polish flag in my room! My wife and I collected Christmas ornaments from each of the places we visited and enjoyed decorating our Christmas tree with the ornaments!
	I very much enjoy Slavic foods (stuffed cabbage and pierogies) and German cuisine (wurst and sauerbraten) as well as Chinese food.
	I am not fond of Mexican food, or of fried chicken.
	Movie interests:
	I love Charlie Chan, and Charlie Chaplin movies, as well as other silent movies.
	My favorite actor is Humphrey Bogart, and favorite movie is "Casablanca."
	I do not enjoy movies with a lot of violence in them.

Domain	Martin's Responses to Key Questions
	Authors of interest: My favorite books to read are biographies. I also like Stephen King novels. During long car rides I enjoy listening to books on tape. I have not used a Kindle or any other electronic devices. *Games of interest:* Games that I enjoy playing include Scrabble and cribbage. *Computer literacy:* I am computer literate and have worked with computers since 1965. My e-mail address is: goodolguy@yahoo.com. I have a webcam, which was set up to communicate with my grandchildren overseas. *Organizational affiliation:* I have been an active member of the Boy Scouts for over 60 years. In addition, I am a lifetime member of the Knights of Columbus, and a fourth degree knight. I have also been a member of the Horticultural Society for over the past 50 years. I also belong to the Pioneer Network of America, a community service organization with membership from retired telephone system employees. The Telephone Pioneers of America presented me with a lifetime achievement award. Other organizations in which I have retained membership include the Knights of Columbus, Kiwanis and Rotary Clubs. *Civic engagement:* I served on our local county boards and held appointed roles in service-related organizations.
Intellectual	*Education:* Initially I completed high school, but during my years working at the telephone company I returned to school and earned a bachelor's degree in accounting, as well as an engineering degree. When I was in my early 50s I also earned an MBA. I have numerous certificates from short courses I took. This also includes work with Six Sigma (I earned a black belt and am a master level Kaizon trainer). *Academic accomplishments:* I was the class valedictorian and received the Lieutenant Governor's medal for academic achievement during my MBA program. *Languages:* I learned to speak English, French, German, Polish, and Russian during my lifetime, and I can also read and write technically in these languages.
Spirituality	*Religious background/history:* I was baptized as an infant into the Catholic faith, and have remained Catholic my entire life.

(continued)

TABLE 13.2 Sample Personal Preference Inventory for "Martin" (*continued*)

Domain	Martin's Responses to Key Questions
	Spiritual practices: I pray the Rosary daily, and I do not eat meat on Fridays. Even though eating meat is now permissible on Fridays, except during Lent, I still like to abstain on Fridays. As I grow older, I would like to continue receive the sacraments, attend a bible study class, and be able to practice my Catholic faith. I would also like to attend Mass on a weekly basis. *Favorite religious celebrations or holidays:* My favorite celebration is Christmas. My wife would always bake wonderful Christmas cookies, and we would have a traditional Polish Christmas Eve dinner. *What are some treasured memories about your spiritual/religious background?* Christmas and Easter traditions are am important part of my spirituality. Our family also celebrated Passover and Hanukkah. We say a blessing over our food prior to every meal.
Physical/ well-being	*Physical health and values about staying healthy:* For most of my life I enjoyed a high-protein, low-carbohydrate diet. Periodically, I do like to fast and drink only water for an entire day.
Mental vitality	*Mental vitality and values about mental vitality:* Meditation and daily prayer help me maintain a balance and preserve my mental vitality. *Health history:* Nothing here to note or record.

ADVOCACY

Advocacy efforts on the part of the individual and his or her family are important strategies to help facilitate resident input and to help support the resident's and family's desire to work toward person-centered planning and a culture change environment. Residents also can exercise their opportunity for advocacy efforts through the resident council meetings. Although resident council meetings may seem daunting to residents who may have not previously participated in any formalized or structured activities, this strategy can be exceedingly helpful in reaching the goal of personal and group advocacy.

The resident council is considered the residents' voice in long-term care facilities. It includes a leadership structure (president or chairperson, vice president or vice chairperson, and secretary). The resident council can also be effective in hiring decisions of care staff and the administrative staff.

FAMILY AND CONSUMER PARTICIPATION

Family participation is also considered an important component of the process of collaborative efforts. Family members have the opportunity to participate in many different committees within the facility but often feel intimidated about participation. Their participation, however, can provide important insight for helping professionals who may not necessarily take into consideration the resident or family perspectives on issues. Usually the social worker, or activities director, can be of assistance when developing linkages for family members to participate as advocates within facility committees.

BUILDING BRIDGES TO FACILITATE PARTICIPATION

If you are reading this chapter because you are currently working in a long-term care facility, the notion of working to build bridges to facilitate participation between a resident and the care providers within the facility may be an idea that has not captured your attention in the past, or an idea that you have not considered very carefully. Each worker has a responsibility to try to build bridges with family members and residents in an effort to recognize those individuals as an integral part of the care team. At times, the process may be challenging and feel out of control. It is important to recognize that residents and family may act in the manner that they do because they do not feel in control of the situation and want to be heard in some positive manner. Building partnerships is a two-way street and requires the active participation of all parties, including the family, the resident, and the care team.

SUMMARY

This chapter explored the role that family and consumer advocates can play in the culture change process. The integration of a PPI into a resident's care plan can help caregivers better understand the individual resident and facilitate a more person-centered care approach. Building partnerships with residents and their families will add their voice to the process of care management and push the internal culture of the facility from one of care to one of "home." This chapter has provided an overview of the importance these partners play in the overall care process and has showcased how to integrate these partners into the process.

DISCUSSION/REFLECTION QUESTIONS

1. What role do families and residents play in the care management partnership for people living in long-term care settings?
2. Develop a PPI for yourself using the guidelines provided. Share this profile with someone close to you, or someone whom you feel knows you well. Was that person surprised at the breadth of information or understanding given in your PPI? Did that person's perception and understanding of you change in any way once he or she knew more about you as a person?
3. Are there some strategies that you can implement to better integrate the voice of residents and families within your facility or setting?

REFERENCES

Andonian, L., & MacRae, A. (2011). Well older adults within an urban context: Strategies to create and maintain social participation. *British Journal of Occupational Therapy, 74,* 2–11.

Braddock, D. (1992). Community mental health and mental retardation services in the United States: A comparative study of resource allocation. *American Journal of Psychiatry, 149,* 175–183.

Heller, T., Petterson, B., & Miller, A. (1996). Guidelines from the consumer: Improving consumer involvement in research and training for persons with mental retardation. *Mental Retardation, 34,* 141–148.

Itzhaky, H., & York, A. S. (1991). Client participation and the effectiveness of community social work interventions. *Research on Social Work Practice, 1*(4), 387–398.

Jurkowski, E. T. (1997). *Leadership/citizen participation in resource planning/development for people with physical disabilities.* Ann Arbor, MI: Dissertation Abstracts International. (Accession number 8676280)

Jurkowski, E. T., Jovanovic, B., & Rowitz, L. (2002). Leadership/citizen participation: Perceived impact of advocacy activities by people with physical disabilities on access to health care, attendant care and social services. *Journal of Health & Social Policy, 14*(4), 49–60.

Keys, C., & Foster-Fishman, P. (2000). Advocacy in the United States: Content and process. In B. Stratford & T. D. Young (Eds.), *Mental retardation: The way ahead.* Hong Kong: Hong Kong Association for the Scientific Study of Mental Handicap.

Lord, J. (1987). The voice of the people: Qualitative research and the needs of consumers. *Canadian Journal of Mental Health, 6*(2), 35–36.

Miller, A., & Keys, C. (1996). The self-advocacy movement for persons with developmental disabilities: Principles of empowerment. *Mental Retardation, 34*(5), 312–319.

Soliman, B. B. (1976). *Black empowerment social work in oppressed communities.* New York, NY: Columbia University Press.

Zimmerman, M. A., & Rappaport, J. (1988). Citizen participation, perceived control and psychological empowerment. *American Journal of Community Psychology, 16*(5), 725–750.

14

Building Coalitions of Effective Change Agent Teams

Coalitions have been powerful vehicles for advocacy, education, knowledge transfer, dissemination, and resource and policy development. They also have been helpful in the development of a tremendous number of initiatives in the arenas of disability and aging. This chapter addresses the dynamics of coalitions and working groups; explores how they have been helpful in a variety of movements, such as the independent-living movement and the culture change movement; and provides a framework for building and sustaining successful coalitions. The chapter concludes with an exploration of specific coalitions available to transform cultures of care.

COALITIONS AND COALITION BUILDING

Coalitions, defined as temporary alliances or factions that can be used in the process of pursuing a political strategy or goal (Jurkowski, 2008), do not evolve without some strategic input from facilitators or individuals skilled with group dynamics in a leadership capacity. In essence, a coalition comprises an organized group of people who are interested in working toward a common goal (Jurkowski, 2008). Coalitions share a common vision, mission, and responsibility along with buy-in from a variety of sectors (The Abraham Lincoln Center for Character Development, 2008). The pioneering movement has mobilized successful coalitions in nearly all of the 50 states. Although officials in each state oversee the development and activities of the coalitions within their state, coalitions exist within regional areas to work for the betterment of long-term care providers across a variety of sectors within the long-term care continuum.

The development of coalitions is predicated on a common vision, mission, and set of goals. Generally speaking, pioneer coalitions have been developed to help promote and foster support for the concept of the pioneering and culture change movement. The goals of these coalitions include the promotion of the person-centered care approach to patient care, fostering the use of the Artifacts of Culture Change Tool (Schoeneman & Bowman, 2006), and advocating for revised policies at the federal and state levels. The ultimate goal of these coalitions is to bring about broad, significant changes in the long-term care movement.

Pioneering network coalitions also can be useful in bringing about a more effective and efficient delivery of care resources to people living in long-term care settings as well as in increasing communication between groups (e.g., the medical community, the long-term care community, and consumers). They can also be helpful in trying to erode stereotypes. Last, coalitions also can be helpful in facilitating social change (Foster, n.d.-a).

Up to this point, the chapter has discussed coalitions as unified entities with all members interested in the same goal. Some political coalitions really are alliances between individuals who represent different interests but who band together to support each other for the sake of seeking a specific resolution or outcome. It is important to understand this kind of coalition because such political alliances can be useful when seeking policy or legislative changes and/or seeking political support to bring a specific issue to attention.

Building effective coalitions, regardless of the reason, requires a number of key components and some specific strategies. An understanding of the dynamics of groups and coalitions is one thing that contributes to effective coalitions. Mobilizing the various components of coalitions, such as key stakeholders, interests, and resources; membership agendas; and mission, vision, and sustainability, contribute to a coalition's success. Each of these components is addressed in the remainder of this chapter. This will help readers understand how to use these components within the process of building their own coalitions.

DYNAMICS OF GROUPS AND COALITIONS

The very process of working with coalitions suggests that groups of people are involved. Thus, as with any group, dynamics are involved. These dynamics are created through the interactions among group members, the interests they bring to the table, and their reactions to specific issues. Factors that influence roles include the needs of specific members within a group, as well as the culture and environment of the group (Jurkowski, 2008).

Any group, regardless of size and purpose, generally will have within its membership three specific types of members: (a) the task-oriented members, (b) the group- or process-oriented members, and (c) the distracters. Each type contributes to the overall culture and progress of the coalition or group. For example, if all members are task oriented, they may not recognize some of the underlying issues that are affecting people within the group. If all members are process oriented, they may spend all their time processing and discussing the emotional side of the members and not ever accomplish any goals or work toward the plan the membership has outlined. If all members have their own agenda, and are not working toward a common goal, the group may be not only dysfunctional but also highly distraction oriented.

These same issues may be common and active within a long-term care facility or home as staff and administrators try to implement the benchmarks discussed in Part II of this book. If the staff are all task oriented, they may not take time to reflect on, or seek input from, residents about their perceptions. For example, does the individual resident feel less lonely, more hopeful, and more connected to others? In a task-centered environment, the focus may be on ensuring the care needs are met, and "checked off the list" for the day. Staff may think that they are offering services in a manner that is person centered; however, listening to feelings and reactions may lead them to a different conclusion.

In a similar way, the individual or environment that is very process oriented could easily run the risk of getting overly engaged in how the benchmarks are being implemented. Ongoing discussions with residents and among staff may result in staff never accomplishing the required resident care needs and a consequent backlog of work. It is important to keep these roles in mind and develop some balance between the two roles in any given setting or team.

Distracters, or people with individual agendas, may also be a threat to the process. Members who fall into this category may interested not in participating in the process but in blocking it. If one considers a hypothetical residential facility, people who are distracters may be the director or administrator who does not want to implement changes to the current status quo, and such an individual's behavior or attitude will influence the implementation and lead to unsuccessful outcomes.

The three roles and their impact are discussed in greater length in the following section.

COMPONENTS OF COALITIONS

Key Stakeholders, Interests, and Resources

Within every coalition, key stakeholders exist, along with their interests and the resources that they bring to the table. In a coalition that is working toward the promotion of person-centered practices, the key stakeholders may include representatives from local area agencies on aging, administrators of long-term care facilities, directors of nursing from long-term care facilities, representatives from the hospice community, family members, marketing representatives from long-term care facilities, care staff (from nursing staff to certified nursing assistants), academics, and service providers. Each may represent a specific set of vested interests, such as marketing and recruitment, service provision, and evaluation of programs and services.

Working with coalitions can also prove challenging, because people in a coalition often represent a host of different interests and agendas. A key factor is to understand the specific interests each key stakeholder may have and understand how the stakeholders represent their interests. Success in managing these various divergent viewpoints can often be linked to building an inventory of each key stakeholder's interests and resources. In this process, managing the various stakeholders can prove to be challenging, but by identifying the specific interests of each organization and individual, one can quickly begin to develop an understanding of why people have become involved in the coalition. In fact, if several people have become involved for the same reason, they may want to work together on a subcommittee or small group to help build strength in their ability to get things done and build a coalition of interests.

Stakeholders also bring resources to coalition efforts. These resources can be tangible or intangible: skills, experiences, energy, social networks, infrastructure, or supplies. Too often people neglect to inventory what resources stakeholders can bring to the table or situation. Without an inventory and an understanding of which resources stakeholders can bring to a situation, coalition groups may find that their progress is stifled or impaired.

One way to build an inventory of stakeholder resources would be to survey members when they attend specific functions and/or survey people when they join advisory groups. Some of the specific items to include on this resource inventory can include areas of expertise (accounting, legal, marketing, computer, research, event planning, fundraising and grant writing, organizational development, resource development, and artwork), networks, and education.

Membership: Group Roles and Responsibilities

Earlier, this chapter addressed the various roles played by members of a coalition; now, this section delves into these roles in an effort to help explain how some specific roles play into the development of coalitions. Table 14.1 outlines some of the specific roles found within coalitions, categorizes what the roles are, and provides a short definition of each role.

TABLE 14.1 An Overview of Coalition Member Roles

Role	Type	Definition	Example
Spokesperson	Task	The spokesperson is responsible for voicing the group's concerns to the coalition or other reference group.	Phil, a consumer on a resident council for the Highlands North West Home, brings the home's concerns following a resident discussion to management of the facility and the Colorado North West Coalition.
Negotiator	Task	The negotiator helps develop alternatives that are "win–win" and attempts to build a consensus among groups with divergent ideas.	The certified nurse assistants and the director of nursing had very different viewpoints on building a person-centered care bathing system. The negotiator in the group was able to bridge the director of nursing's concerns regarding time management with the certified nurse assistants' concerns regarding timing of baths/spas.
Advocate	Task	The advocate speaks up to represent the group's interests. He or she usually strives to represent interests that are consistent with the group's mission.	When new management took over the Desoto Nursing Facility and wanted to do away with consistent nursing assignments with residents, the resident council president advocated for the importance of consistent assignments.

(continued)

TABLE 14.1 An Overview of Coalition Member Roles (*continued*)

Role	Type	Definition	Example
Initiator	Task	The initiator will begin the process of voicing concerns.	Bill, Jane's cousin, who volunteers on the resident advisory board, promptly voices concerns about restrictions to resident autonomy and supported Jane in her quest for computer webcam access in the facility's library.
Organizer	Task	The organizer takes charge of projects or committees. This person generally has strong delegation skills.	Mark is quick to make committee assignments at the pioneer steering committee meetings.
Consultant	Task	The consultant has expertise in a specific area of interest to the group and provides advice as needed.	Meagan provides consultant advice for cosmetic changes to the environment. She enjoys using her skills, which she acquired while studying interior design.
Contributor	Task	The contributor provides information or data that will help advance the mission of the group.	Richard, the regional director for the CA Department of Public Health, is consistently sharing data from the health department on citations and accompanying solutions for regulatory code violations to the pioneer coalition advisory board and coalition members.
Information seeker	Task	The information seeker will seek out alternative sources of information that will help in the decision-making process.	Samantha used the contacts in Appendix B to find out how other pioneering coalitions across the nation were handling changes to Medicare regulations.
Opinion seeker	Task	The opinion seeker makes no secret of facilitating what group members think about a project or initiative set forward by the group/mission/vision.	John made it a point to ask for feedback on new policy directions from all board members.
Energizer	Task	The energizer provides the strength to carry on and helps invigorate members of the advisory group or coalition to meet some common goals.	Consistently, at coalition training meetings, Todd presents his mascot and song to encourage members to carry out the coalition's person-centered care mission and vision.

Role	Type	Definition	Example
Encourager	Group process	The encourager helps members who are on the fringe or sidelines remain involved.	Martha will begin an hour before resident council meetings, trying to recruit participants from the household to participate in the monthly meetings.
Harmonizer	Group process	The harmonizer ensures that there is balance among membership.	Jillian always tries to ensure that both task-oriented and process-oriented members have an opportunity to participate.
Gatekeeper	Group process	The gatekeeper helps keep the channels of communication open.	Theresa is always actively listening and trying to paraphrase statements to try to ensure that the conservative and liberal viewpoints on the committee are heard, valued, and respected.
Standard setter	Group process	The standard setter helps people remain true to the benchmarks that have been established.	Cinda plays the role of the standard setter within the pioneer collaborative to ensure that all facilities are aspiring to meet their benchmarks identified in the Artifacts of Culture Change Assessment Tool.
Group observer	Group process	The group observer provides watch over the group to observe specific group dynamics.	Sydney and Lisa have been assigned the roles on the board to ensure that communication flows and to identify what roles members play and which players take on task versus group process roles.
Follower	Group process	The follower goes with the flow and does not challenge the process or interfere or create roadblocks to success.	Tobias, Emily, and Martha consistently attend Pioneer Network meetings but are passive participants. They rarely participate in discussions, never present, conflict and always vote with the majority.

Some of the specific roles in coalitions that are task oriented include the roles of initiator, negotiator, advocate, spokesperson, organizer, consultant, contributor, information seeker, opinion seeker, and energizer. Roles that are process oriented include the encourager, harmonizer, gatekeeper, standard setter, group observer, and follower. Each of these roles provides some unique contributions to the coalition's success and the efforts it is trying to promote, especially, for example, pioneering coalitions.

Agendas

An agenda is basically the purpose for being and doing what a group is given the responsibility to carry out. Individual and group agendas are always going to be present in any group or coalition. The key to a successful coalition, however, is to ensure that key stakeholders and members are committed to a common agenda. This agenda can be reflected in the group's mission and vision. In addition, meetings should always have a drafted set of items to be discussed and deliberated on, which will also take the form of an agenda.

Mission

Mission statements lay out the purpose and goal of any organization or entity. Coalition groups function best with a clear mission that has been embraced by key stakeholders. During the formation stage of a coalition group, a mission statement needs to be affirmed. This process will then support ongoing efforts to meet the mission.

Vision

A common vision, or purpose, is a key component of a successful coalition. An unclear idea of the big picture, or what the coalition is working toward, can lead to rudderless travel. Effective coalitions keep a common vision in place to ensure a common purpose among its membership. One way to help promote this common vision is to have frequent reminders of what the vision is, and use the vision to help brand the coalition. The vision or purpose of the coalition can be revisited at meetings, and all correspondence from the advisory group or leadership can include a "sound bite" with a few words that help promote the vision. For example, a coalition formed to promote the values of The Pioneering Network could use a message that would reads "Promoting and supporting quality care" on all newsletters and correspondence.

Sustainability

The last of the components of coalitions that this chapter discusses is sustainability. All too often, coalitions do not sustain their energy and enthusiasm because people fail to see progress or fail to feel that their involvement and engagement make a difference. A few strategies can help cultivate engagement and help sustain efforts. These include recognition, building a climate of respect, creating meaningful roles for members within coalitions, cultivating relationships among members, building rewards for membership, and demonstrating results (Kaye, 2012).

Recognition is key for membership within any organization or coalition. People are more likely to continue participating in specific organizations and coalitions if they feel that their efforts are recognized and supported. One form of recognition involves public praise and awards. Participation awards that target volunteers and key stakeholders help sustain the members' energy and involvement. One's efforts can also be recognized at public events, through communications, and at specific recognition dinners. Printed certificates of acknowledgment for stakeholder and volunteer efforts are also small but significant ways to offer rewards for leadership and stakeholder/volunteer involvement.

A second key element to sustainability is a climate of respect. Coalition members, as well as key stakeholders, need to feel that they are respected and their time is valued. Scheduling time to meet can be an issue, in particular if meetings are held during the daytime when people are working. On the other hand, professionals who are part of stakeholder groups may not be able, or want, to attend evening meetings. The key is to be able to accommodate most people's needs in regard to when to meet, or to hold meetings on alternate days to meet most people's schedules. Differing values, and ethnic and professional cultures, also play a role in member and stakeholder perceptions. These will influence how people relate to each other and how they react to decision making. Within the myriad reactions, keep in mind that people genuinely always need to feel respected and valued.

A third factor that can impact the sustainability of a coalition involves the importance of meaningful roles. Each member and/or stakeholder should feel like his or her contribution and input have some significant bearing on the outcome and mission of the coalition. Too often, residents and family members, although vital to the process, feel like they cannot contribute to the discussions or major questions. Neither members nor stakeholders should be made to feel like they are "tokens" within any capacity, and their input should be given the same value as their peers.

Cultivating relationships among the networks is also an important factor in the sustainability of a coalition. These relationships include those between members and between organizations. Opportunities for both networking and for relationships between members and/or stakeholders must exist. If the members/stakeholders within the coalition feel like they are strangers to one another, then no sense of cohesiveness will exist between them (Foster, n.d.-b).

Building rewards for members of the coalition and key stakeholders will also help sustain coalitions. Rewards may be tangible, such as recognition certificates and public recognition ceremonies, or intangible, such as resources and information, networking, access to people in decision-making capacities, or affluence and social time. A couple of examples to help illustrate these points include the use of affluence when a local legislator comes to visit a local long-term care facility and meet with resident representatives to hear their concerns through a fireside chat. Additional social time can include a field trip to the local shopping mall or a lunch out at a resident's favorite restaurant.

A final key factor for sustainability is demonstrable results. Organizational effectiveness and clear accomplishments are a solid way to attract people and help ensure that they will want to be an active part of mobilizing the organization. A definite strategy to influence sustainability is to create visible and ongoing successes.

ADVANCES IN THE DISABILITY AND AGING MOVEMENTS THROUGH COALITIONS

Coalitions have been responsible for advances within the arenas of both disability and aging. Most notably, the passage of the Americans with Disabilities Act of 1990 (ADA) can be attributed to the work of disability-oriented coalition groups across the United States (Jurkowski, 2008). A version of the ADA was set forward as a bill to the Congress and the Senate in the late 1980s; however, disability rights advocacy groups did not support each other and engage in a common mission and vision in relation to the passage of the legislation. Support and advocacy efforts were not consistent from state to state, or from interest group to interest group. After the unsuccessful outcome of the originally proposed ADA, the Coalition of Disability Rights Organizations was formed, with a mission to work together and provide legislative advocacy. Disability rights groups across a range of sectors carried out a united front in terms of mission and vision and conveyed a consistent message to legislators regarding the passage of the proposed legislation. Regardless of state or counties within individual states, the message was consistent as a result of the coalition. The end result was the successful passage of the 1990 ADA. The ADA benefits both people with disabilities, as well as people growing older who have mobility and sensory impairments.

THE PIONEER NETWORK AND COALITIONS

Currently, coalitions promoting the work of the pioneer movement exist at least throughout the United States and Canada. Within the United States there is a national office with dedicated resources to help foster coalitions throughout the country. Several states have statewide offices that provide services and resources to coalitions within the state, whereas some states have only some organized coalitions within local communities. Regardless of the organizational approaches, the concept of coalitions to promote the work of the Pioneer Network is thriving and will probably be one of the key elements in fostering the mission and changing the culture of long-term care in the future. A detailed list of coalitions and contacts for these entities are available in Appendix A.

A CHECKLIST FOR ESTABLISHING AND FOSTERING A COALITION

Checklists can be useful tools in the day-to-day work of professionals who are trying to develop a plan or organizational framework. In a similar way, checklists can be used to help identify priorities in planning for coalition efforts and periodically evaluating the impact and health of the coalition.

If you and/or your organization are in the initial stages of organizing and cultivating energies to build a coalition, the issues of course will be quite different than when evaluating the relative success or health of a coalition. When beginning to develop partners for a coalition, identify the care providers in your target community for which you want to develop your coalition. Building a contact list will be an important tool, especially when trying to maintain communication. In addition, consider building an e-mail and telephone text database of all potential members, because these will become major venues for communication.

Set up an advisory board to assist with the planning and implementation of specific collation activities. Consider, within this advisory board, potential members and the skills they can bring to the table to help build and support the coalition. Some of the professional areas where skill development can be an asset include computer skills; fund-raising skills/development; and expertise in event planning, grant writing, legislation and policy affairs, marketing, legal issues, media relations, training/teaching, research, writing and editing, and organizational management. The advisory board will be helpful in shaping the direction and activities of the coalition. When trying to recruit board members, it may also be helpful to have some specific job descriptions and an explanation of time commitment. In today's active society, people may be very guarded about how they want to provide a time commitment without a clear understanding of what their new roles would entail.

Once the structural components are in place, the advisory board and coalition members personalize and tailor the activities for the coalition. Identify a clear mission and develop support through consensus from members of the advisory board and membership. Based on the mission, identify some goals and objectives with some clear benchmarks. A strategic plan can also be helpful in orchestrating activities; however, it may be more fruitful to identify a timeline for accomplishing goals and objectives. Keep in mind that it is very helpful to have a periodic review of the goals and objectives and evaluate the extent to which these have been mastered, or whether additional time and resources are needed. Periodic review, evaluation, and discussion about what resources are needed, and what resources should be restructured and reinvented, is a critical element for the success of coalitions (Erkowitz & Schultz, n.d.). Table 14.2 provides a checklist to help with developing a coalition.

Periodic evaluation of the coalition and its effectiveness also is important. Griffen (2000) provided a short questionnaire/checklist to help coalitions examine their impact and effectiveness. Items on the checklist include community and political support, diversity, membership decision making, leadership, communication, and resources. Table 14.3 provides a sample checklist to help evaluate a coalition's effectiveness.

TABLE 14.2 Checklist for Establishing a Coalition

Activity	Person Responsible	Date Assigned	Target Completion	Follow-Up
Develop a contact list of all providers within the target area.				
Build an electronic database for membership, including an e-mail and telephone text database.				
Develop an inventory of potential competencies and experts who can provide some expertise and support to an advisory board.				
Develop an advisory board.				
Build job descriptions for various activities within the advisory board and coalitions.				
Develop a mission statement for the coalition.				
Develop some goals and objectives to be accomplished.				
Establish a timeline for establishing the goals and objectives.				

Table 14.3 A Checklist for Evaluating Coalition Effectiveness

Time Period 1	Time Period 2	Item	Strongly Agree (4)	Agree (3)	Disagree (2)	Strongly Disagree (1)	Unsure (0)
		1. Community and political support exists for the work of the coalition.					
		2. Membership within the coalition represents a range of sectors within the community.					
		3. Diverse sectors of the community are represented within coalition membership.					
		4. There is strong leadership representing and leading our coalition.					
		5. There is frequent and regular communication with the broader community.					
		6. We have sufficient resources to achieve our goals.					

(continued)

Table 14.3 A Checklist for Evaluating Coalition Effectiveness (continued)

Time Period 1	Time Period 2	Item	Strongly Agree (4)	Agree (3)	Disagree (2)	Strongly Disagree (1)	Unsure (0)
		7. The vision and goals of our coalition are clear and commonly understood.					
		8. The process of making decisions is clear and inclusive.					
		9. We celebrate our successes.					
		10. Are there steps that we could take in the next 6 months to improve the effectiveness of our coalition? Yes No (Circle one) Explanation:					
		11. What are three steps we could take within the next 6 months to improve the effectiveness of our coalition? A. B. C.					

(Adapted from Griffin, 2000.)

SUMMARY

This chapter reviewed the concept of coalitions and showcased some of the steps in building effective coalitions, especially in the case of pioneer coalitions. The chapter also reviewed the concept of coalitions and coalition building and outlined how coalitions can be helpful in furthering the mission of the culture change framework. The specific dynamics that influence groups and communities were showcased and discussed. Components of effective coalitions have been reviewed and articulated. The Pioneer Network and pioneering coalitions have been reviewed, and a checklist for building and sustaining effective coalitions was provided.

DISCUSSION/REFLECTION QUESTIONS

1. Identify a local pioneer coalition that exists in your area. Attend a meeting and identify what the group's current activities, goals, and objectives may be. Could you get involved in the coalition in some way and, if so, how do you envision your involvement?
2. If a local coalition is not available, use Table 14.1 to begin to identify, with other stakeholders, what steps would be important to walk through to develop one.
3. Using the checklist in Table 14.2, visit with the chairperson of a coalition in your area and interview him or her regarding his or her coalition. Using the findings from your interview, prepare a short report and recommendations that can be shared back with the group.

REFERENCES

The Abraham Lincoln Center for Character Development. (2008). *Coalition building*. Retrieved from http://www.lincolncharacter.org/cdc-coalition.htm

Erkowitz, B., & Schultz, J. (n.d.). *Coalition building: Starting a coalition*. New York, NY: GLSEN Field Development Resources.

Foster, D. (n.d.-a). *Coalition planning*. Amherst, MA: AHEC/Community Partners.

Foster, D. (n.d.-b). *Engaging residents in coalition building*. Amherst, MA: AHEC/Community Partners.

Griffin, G. (2000). Coalition effectiveness: How are we doing?

Jurkowski, E. T. (2008). *Policy and program planning for older adults: Realities and visions*. New York, NY: Springer Publishing.

Kaye, G. (2012). *The six R's of participation*. Amherst, MA: AHEC/Community Partners.

Schoeneman, K., & Bowman, C. (2006). *Development of the artifacts of culture change tool: Report of contract HHSM-500-2005-00076P* (technical report). Baltimore, MD: Centers for Medicaid & Medicare Services. Retrieved from http://www.artifactsofculturechange.org/Data/Documents/artifacts.pdf

15

Legal and Regulatory Bodies and the Culture Change Process

Transforming the paradigm of thinking and the organizational practices associated with these paradigms can be a challenge at best. Layering on the legal and regulatory expectations that may also need to be addressed may be the impetus for an organization to maintain a tight grip on their initial paradigm. The shift to a culture change paradigm can be threating for long-term care facilities, simply because of the fear that mandated regulations may not be followed appropriately or consistently. Establishing new benchmarks for practice in long-term care settings can elicit similar feelings of threat and discomfort.

The purpose of this chapter is to explore a specific set of benchmark arenas and identify strategies that long-term care facilities may be able to use to address the regulatory mandates. The chapter concludes with some tips for working with state and federal regulatory bodies to help pave the way for transformation into a paradigm of culture change and a renewed set of benchmarks for practice within one's long-term care setting. The following pages of interpretive guidelines were reprinted from a memo crafted by the Centers for Medicare & Medicaid (2012).

Rather than trying to reinterpret the material, it has been reprinted here without rewording of the explanations in many instances.

CARE PRACTICES: DIGNITY OF THE INDIVIDUAL

F241 Dignity

483.15(a) Dignity

> The facility must promote care for residents in a manner and in an environment that maintains or enhances each resident's dignity and respect in full recognition of his or her individuality.

Interpretive Guidelines
"Dignity" means that in their interactions with residents, staff carries out activities that assist the resident to maintain and enhance his or her self-esteem and self-worth. Some examples include (but are not limited to):

- *Maintaining an environment in which there are no signs posted in residents' rooms or in staff work areas able to be seen by other residents and/or visitors that include confidential clinical or personal information (such as information about incontinence, cognitive status). It is allowable to post signs with this type of information in more private locations such as the inside of a closet or in staff locations that are not viewable by the public. An exception can be made in an individual case if a resident or responsible family member insists on the posting of care information at the bedside (e.g., do not take blood pressure in right arm). This does not prohibit the display of resident names on their doors nor does it prohibit display of resident memorabilia and/or biographical information in or outside their rooms with their consent or the consent of the responsible party if the resident is unable to give consent. (This restriction does not include the [Centers for Disease Control and Prevention] isolation precaution transmission-based signage for reason of public health protection, as long as the sign does not reveal the type of infection).*

SELF-DETERMINATION AND PARTICIPATION

F242 Self-Determination and Participation

483.15(b) Self-Determination and Participation

> The resident has the right to—
> 1. Choose activities, schedules, and health care consistent with his or her interests, assessments, and plans of care;
> 2. Interact with members of the community both inside and outside the facility; and
> 3. Make choices about aspects of his or her life in the facility that is significant to the resident.

The intent of this requirement is to specify that the facility must create an environment that is respectful of the right of each resident to exercise his or her autonomy regarding what the resident considers to be important facets of his or her life. *This includes actively seeking information from the resident regarding significant interests and preferences in order to provide necessary assistance to help residents fulfill their choices over aspects of their lives in the facility.*

Many types of choices are mentioned in this regulatory requirement. The first of these is choice over "activities." It is an important right for a resident to have choices to participate in preferred activities, whether they are part of the formal activities program or self-directed.

PERSON FIRST NEEDS

F246 Accommodation of Needs

483.15(e) Accommodation of Needs

> A resident has the right to reside and receive services in the facility with reasonable accommodation of individual needs and preferences, except when the health or safety of the individual or other residents would be endangered.

Interpretive Guidelines: 483.15(e)(1)
"Reasonable accommodations of individual needs and preferences" means the facility's efforts to individualize the resident's *physical* environment. *This includes the physical environment of the resident's bedroom and bathroom, as well as individualizing as much as feasible the facility's common living areas.* The facility's physical environment and staff behaviors should be directed toward assisting the resident in maintaining and/or achieving independent functioning, dignity, and well-being to the extent possible in accordance with the resident's own *needs and* preferences.

The facility is responsible for evaluating each resident's unique needs and preferences and ensuring that the environment accommodates the resident to the extent reasonable and does not endanger the health or safety of individuals or other residents. This includes making adaptations of the resident's bedroom and bathroom furniture and fixtures as necessary to ensure that the resident can (if able):

- *Open and close drawers and turn faucets on and off;*
- *See her/himself in a mirror and have toiletry articles easily within reach while using the sink;*
- *Open and close bedroom and bathroom doors, easily access areas of their room and bath, and operate lighting;*
- *Use bathroom facilities as independently as possible with access to assistive devices (such as grab bars within reach) if needed; and*
- *Perform other desired tasks such as turning a table light on and off, using the call bell; and so on.*

NOTE: *If a resident cannot reach her/his clothing in the closet, if the resident does not have private closet space, or if the resident does not have needed furniture (such as a chair) refer to 483.15(h)(4) and 483.70(d)(2)(iv). F461.*

The facility should strive to provide reasonable sufficient electric outlets to accommodate the resident's need to safely use her/his electronic personal items, as long as caution is maintained to not overload circuits. The bedroom should include comfortable seating for the resident and should accommodate the resident's preferences for arrangement of furniture to the extent space allows, including facilitating resident choice about where to place their bed in their room (as long as the roommate, if any, concurs). There may be some limitations on furniture arrangement, such as not placing a bed over a heat register, or not placing a bed far from the call cord so as to make it unreachable from the bedside.

The facility should also ensure that furniture and fixtures in common areas frequented by resident are accommodating of physical limitations of residents. Furnishings in common areas should enhance residents' abilities to maintain their independence, such as being able to arise from living room furniture. The facility should provide seating with appropriate seat height, of accommodating residents of different heights and differing types of needs in common areas is through the use of different sizes and types of furniture.

NOTE: If residents are prohibited from using common area restrooms, the lobby, or dining rooms outside of meal times, refer to 483.15(a), F241, Dignity. For issues of sufficient lighting, refer to 483.15(h)(5), F256, Adequate and Comfortable Lighting.

Staff should strive to reasonably accommodate the resident's needs and preferences as the resident makes use of the physical environment. This includes ensuring that items the resident needs to use are available and accessible to encourage confidence and independence (such as handle grippers) are maintained in place and functional furniture is arranged to accommodate the resident's needs and preferences, and so on. This does not apply to residents who need extensive staff assistance and are incapable of using these room adaptations.

ENVIRONMENT

F252 Environment

483.15(h) Environment

> The facility must provide—
>
> 483.15(h)(1) A safe, clean, comfortable, and homelike environment, allowing the resident to use his or her personal belongings to the extent possible.

Interpretive Guidelines: 483.15(h)(1)
For purposes of this requirement, "environment" refers to any environment in the facility that is frequented by residents, including *(but not limited to)* the residents' rooms, bathrooms, hallways, *dining areas, lobby, outdoor patios,* therapy areas, and activity areas. A determination of "homelike" should include the resident's opinion of the living environment.

A "homelike environment" is one that deemphasizes the institutional character of the setting, to the extent possible, and allows the resident to use those personal belongings that support a homelike environment. A personalized, homelike environment recognizes the individuality and autonomy of the resident, provides an opportunity for self-expression, and encourages links with past and family members. *The intent of the word "homelike" in this regulation is that the nursing home should provide an environment as close to that of the environment of a private home as possible. This concept of creating a home setting includes the elimination of institutional odors, and practices to the extent possible. Some good practices that serve to decrease the institutional character of the environment include the elimination of:*

- *Overhead paging and piped-in music throughout the building;*
- *Meal services in the dining room using trays (some residents may wish to eat certain meals in their rooms on trays);*
- *Institutional signage labeling work rooms/closets in areas visible to residents and the public;*
- *Medication carts (some innovative facilities store medications in locked areas in resident rooms);*
- *The widespread and long-term use of audible (to the resident) chair and bed alarms, instead of their limited use for selected residents for diagnostic purposes or according to their care planned needs. These devices can startle the resident and constrain the resident from normal repositioning movements, which can be problematic. For more information about the detriments of alarms in terms of their effects on residents and alternatives to the widespread use of alarms, see the 2007 CS satellite broadcast training, "From Institutionalized to Individualized Care," part 1, available through the National Technical Information Service and other sources such as the Pioneer Network;*
- *Mass purchased furniture, drapes, and bedspreads that all look alike throughout the building (some innovators invite the placement of some residents' furniture in common areas); and*
- *Large, centrally located nursing/care team stations.*

Many facilities cannot immediately make these types of changes, but it should be a goal for all facilities that have not yet made these types of changes to work toward them. *A nursing facility is not considered non-compliant if it still has some of these institutional features, but the facility is expected to do all it can within fiscal constraints to provide an environment that enhances quality of life for residents, in accordance with resident preferences.*

A "homelike" or homey environment is not achieved simply through enhancements to the physical environment. It concerns striving for person-centered care that emphasizes individualization, relationships, and a psychosocial environment that welcomes each resident and makes her/him comfortable.

In a facility in which most residents come for a short-term stay, the "good practices" listed in this section are just as important as in a facility with a majority of long-term care residents. A resident in the facility for a short-term stay would not typically move her/his bedroom furniture into the room but may desire to bring a television, chair, or other personal belongings to have while staying in the facility.

Although the regulatory language at this tag refers to "safe," "clean," "comfortable," and "homelike," for consistency, the following specific F-tags should be used for certain issues of safety and cleanliness:

- For issues of safety of the environment, presence of hazards and hazardous practices, use 483.25(h), Accidents F323.
- For issues of fire danger, use 483.70(a) Life Safety from Fire F454;
- For issues of cleanliness and maintenance of common living areas frequented by residents, use 484.15(h)(2), Housekeeping and Maintenance F253.
- For issues of cleanliness of areas of the facility used by staff only (e.g., break room, medication room, laundry, kitchen, etc.) or the public only (e.g., parking lot), use 483.70(h) F465 Other Environmental Conditions; and
- Although this tag can be used for issues of general comfortableness of the environment such as furniture, there are more specific Tags to use for the following issues:
  - For issues of uncomfortable lighting use 483.15(h)(5), F256 Adequate and Comfortable Lighting;
  - For issues of uncomfortable temperature use 483.15(h)(6), F257 Comfortable and Safe Temperature Levels; and
  - For issues of uncomfortable noise levels, use 483.15(h)(7), F258 Comfortable Sound Levels.

F256 Environment

483.15(h)(5) Environment

The Facility must provide—

483.15(h)(5) Adequate and comfortable lighting levels in all areas.

Interpretive Guidelines 483.15(h)(5)
"Adequate lighting" means levels of illumination suitable to tasks the resident chooses to perform or the facility staff must perform.

"Comfortable lighting" means lighting that minimizes glare and provides maximum resident control, where feasible, over the intensity, location, and direction of illumination so that visually impaired residents can maintain or enhance independent functioning.

As a person ages, their eyes usually change so that they require more light to see what they are doing and where they are going. An adequate lighting design has these features:

- *Sufficient lighting with minimum glare in areas frequented by residents;*
- *Even light levels in common areas and hallways, avoiding patches of low light caused by too much space between light fixtures, within limits of building design constraints;*
- *Use of daylight as much as possible;*
- *Elimination of high levels of glare produced by shiny flooring and from unshielded window openings (no-shine floor waxes and light filtering curtains help to alleviate these sources of glare);*
- *Extra lighting, such as table and floor lamps, to provide sufficient light to assist residents with tasks such as reading;*
- *Lighting for residents who need to find their way from bed to bathroom at night (e.g., red colored night lights preserve night vision); and*
- *Dimming switches in resident rooms (where possible and when desired by the resident) so that staff can tend to a resident at night with limited disturbances to them or a roommate. If dimming is not feasible, another option may be for staff to use flashlight/pen lights when they provide night care.*

Some facilities may not be able to make some of these changes due to voltage or wiring issues. For more information about adequate lighting design for long-term care facilities, a facility may consult the lighting guidance available from the Illuminating Engineering Society of North American, which provides authoritative minimum lighting guidance.

The following are additional visual enhancements a facility should consider making as fiscal constraints permit in order to make it easier for residents with impaired vision to see and use their environment;

- *Use of contrasting color between flooring and baseboard to enable residents with impaired vision to determine the horizontal plane of the floor;*
- *Use of contrast painting of bathroom walls and/or contrasting colored toilet seats so that residents with impaired vision can distinguish the toilet fixture from the wall; and*

- Use of dishware that contrasts with the table or tablecloth color to aid residents with impaired vision to see their food.

RESIDENT ROOMS/BEDROOMS

F461 Resident Rooms

483.70(d)(1)(vi) Resident Rooms

> Bedrooms must—
>
> 483.70(d)(1)(vi) Have at least one window to the outside.

Interpretive Guidelines 483.70(d)(1)(vi)
A facility with resident room windows, as defined by section 18.3.8 of the 2000 edition of the Life Safety Code, or that open to an atrium in accordance with Life Safety Code can meet this requirement for a window to the outside.

In addition to conforming with the Life Safety Code, this requirement was included to assist the resident's orientation to day and night, weather, and general awareness of space outside the facility. The facility is required to provide for a "safe, clean, comfortable and homelike environment" by deemphasizing the institutional character of the setting, to the extent possible. Windows are an important aspect in assuring the homelike environment of a facility. *The allowable window sill height shall not exceed 36 inches. The window may be operable.*
    483.70(d)(1)(vii) Have a floor at or above grade level.

Interpretive Guidelines 483.70(d)(1)(vii)
"At or above grade level" means a room in which the room floor is at or above the surrounding exterior ground level.

> 483.70(d)(2) The facility must provide each resident with—
>
>   i. A separate bed of proper size and height for the convenience of the resident;
>   ii. A clean, comfortable mattress;
>   iii. Bedding, appropriate to the weather and climate; and
>
> 483.70(d)(2)(iv) Functional furniture appropriate to the resident's needs, and individual closet space in the resident's bedroom with clothes rack and shelves accessible to the resident.

483.15(h)(4) Private closet space in each resident room, as specified in 483.70(d)(2)(iv) of this part;

Interpretive Guidelines: 483.70(d)(2)(iv) and 483.15(h)(4)

"Functional furniture appropriate to the resident's needs" means that the furniture in each resident's room contributes to the resident attaining or maintaining his or her highest practicable level of independence and well-being. In general, furnishings include a place to put clothing away in an organized manner that will let it remain clean, free of wrinkles, and accessible to the resident while protecting it from casual access by others; a place to put personal effects such as pictures and a bedside clock, and furniture suitable for the comfort of the resident and visitors (e.g., a chair).

For issues with arrangement of room furniture according to resident needs and preferences, see 483.15(e) Accommodation of Needs F246.

"Clothes racks and shelves accessible to the resident" means that residents can get to and reach their hanging clothing whenever they choose.

"Private closet space" means that each resident's clothing is kept separate from clothing of roommates(s).

> The term "closet space" is not necessarily limited to a space installed into the wall. For some facilities without such installed closets, compliance may be attained through the use of storage furniture such as wardrobes. Out-of-season items may be stored in alternate locations outside the resident's room.

483.70(d)(3) CMS or in the case of a nursing facility the survey agency, may permit variations in requirements specified in paragraphs (d)(1)(i) and (ii) of this section relating to rooms in individual cases when the facility demonstrates in writing that the variations—

  i. Are in accordance with the special needs of the residents; and
  ii. Will not adversely affect residents' health and safety.

Interpretive Guidelines: 483.70(d)(3)

A variation must be in accordance with the special needs of the residents and must not adversely affect the health or safety of residents. Facility hardship is not part of the basis for granting a variation. Since the special needs of residents may change periodically, or different residents may be transferred into a room that has been granted a variation, variations must be reviewed and considered for renewal whenever the facility is certified. If the needs of the residents within the room have not changed since the last annual inspection, the variance should continue if the facility so desires.

Interpretive Guidelines: 483.70(d)(1)(i)
As residents are transferred or discharged from rooms with more than four residents, beds should be removed from the variance until the number of residents occupying the room does not exceed four.

CALL SYSTEMS

F463 Resident Call System

483.70(f) Resident Call System

> The nurses' station must be equipped to receive resident calls through a communication system from—
>
> 1. Resident rooms; and
> 2. Toilet and bathing facilities

Intent: 483.70(f)
The intent of this requirement is that residents, when in their rooms and toilet and bathing areas, have a means of directly contacting caregivers. In the case of an existing centralized nursing station, this communication may be through audible or visual signals and may include "wireless systems." *In those cases in which a facility has moved to decentralized nurse/care team work areas, the intent may be met through other electronic systems that provide direct communication from the resident to the caregivers.*

Interpretive Guidelines: 483.70
This requirement is met only if all portions of the system are functioning (e.g., system is not turned off at the nurses' station, the volume is too low to be heard, the light above a room or rooms is not working) and calls are being answered. For wireless systems, compliance is met only if staff who answer resident calls have functioning devices in their possession and are answering resident calls.

SUMMARY

This chapter reviewed several F-tags and provided some interpretive guidelines from the Centers for Medicare & Medicaid (2012). Although the most significant components have been discussed in this chapter, they are not exhaustive. Within this chapter, care practices for the dignity of the individual, self-determination and participation, person-first needs, environment, resident rooms/bedrooms, and call systems have all been reviewed. Some interpretive guidelines for building a culture change approach to residential care also were addressed.

DISCUSSION/REFLECTION QUESTIONS

1. *What are some of the interpretive guidelines that surprised you? Which guidelines seem reasonably easy to implement? Which may pose some challenge to implement?*
2. *In your state, which guidelines pose a challenge from the perspective of the Department of Public Health survey team? How could you shift the interpretation of the guideline to become more person centered and oriented toward a culture change philosophy?*
3. *What are some interpretive guidelines that you and/or your facility would like to see developed and implemented that were not included within this chapter? How would you build some verbiage for the interpretive guideline?*

REFERENCE

Centers for Medicare & Medicaid. (2012). *Interpretive guidelines memorandum.* Baltimore, MD: Author.

16

A Vision for the Future

This book has taken us on a journey through the land of culture change. Throughout, readers have been exposed to demographic trends that affect the aging population. The book also explored the history of aging services and long-term care services and then rode through the changes in philosophical paradigms that have shaped the culture change approach to long-term care. From this juncture, the chapters began to explore the work of culture change and the benchmarks that frame the culture change perspective. The culture change movement is about changing not only the way programs and services are delivered, but also the way frail elders are viewed. At one time, elderly people were stripped of their dignity and autonomy upon entry into a long-term care facility and have remained dependent on care, but I am hoping we have turned a corner and have begun to explore ways to shift into a person-centered approach through the principles of the culture change movement.

Chapters 4 through 11 of this book gave readers an orientation to the Artifacts of Culture Change Tool (Schoeneman & Bowman, 2006) and the six domains within it that shape the basis for a culture change approach. Each chapter oriented readers to a different aspect of the culture change domain of care, ranging from the environment, person-centered care practices, family and community practices, workplace practices, leadership, and outcomes. In each chapter, specific benchmarks were reviewed, and readers had the opportunity to glean some best-practice examples of how each benchmark has been addressed in facilities across the United States.

The last section of the book focused on strategies to implement a culture change approach to care. Tools were addressed that are essential in the development and implementation of a culture change approach. These included the assessment process, coalition building, building partnerships with family and community, evaluation approaches, and community building.

CONCLUSION

The culture change paradigm, which has been around for over a decade, is probably, at this point, not a fad but here to stay. The increase in baby boomers and the consumerism perspective toward services and resources that permeate our society will continue to influence our expectations for care as people age. Regardless of the expectations the baby boomer generation has for themselves or their parents, the expectation that this group will continue to have, and the part these expectations will play in the development of resources, will help foster the culture change movement.

DIRECTIONS FOR THE FUTURE

We have only just begun our journey. True culture change would not need coalition forces to continue to promote and advocate for person-centered care and would not require toolkits and guidelines. If we had arrived at the end of our journey, then we probably would have no need for a book on this topic. Each and every reader is charged with the responsibility and enthusiasm to promote the resident first and advocate the concept of person-centered care. However, the job still would not be completed even if we endorsed a person-centered care approach and the benchmarks laid out within this book. Despite the myriad benchmarks, many still remain on the horizon to be addressed if people want to be considered truly autonomous and valued for their self-worth and dignity. Some of the areas that should be considered for the future include a variety of taboo subjects that may accompany people into their long-term care facilities. These issues include the following:

> Substance use and access: People who have chronically used substances as a recreational outlet will expect to continue this lifestyle.
>
> Same-sex relationships and long-term relationships that residents will want to remain intact within the long-term care setting. This will include the need for visiting privileges and an acknowledgment

that both parties are in a consensual relationship, supporting each other's needs.

The need for sex, sensuality, and intimacy within long-term care settings. Keeping this in mind, facilities will be challenged to develop policies and support to help couples, regardless of orientation, remain active sensually in long-term care settings.

Opportunities to meet one's technological lifestyle. As baby boomers settle into long-term care settings, they will want to have the technological capacity to be able to use their technology devices. People will expect to be able to use their iPhones, iPads, and laptops in order to communicate with the outside world. They will also expect that their care planning be a click away, and loaded on their technology devices.

Fantasy-oriented environments: Boomers have grown up with Star Wars, Star Trek, and avatar worlds. This love of science fiction, "Trekkies, or Dr. Who," embraced by Baby Boomers will not end with the finale of a season of television shows, or movies. In fact, this affiliation will probably find a transition into long-term care settings.

Services and resources to meet the growing health challenges. As the fields of science and medicine have evolved, so too have the resources available to help promote quality of life and to sustain life. The workforce, families, and consumers will be challenged with ethical dilemmas related to the quality of their life or face choices about sustaining life through artificial strategies and interventions.

In addition to the practice dimensions that require review, the realm of policy development, which will include new ways to craft long-term care policies and implement the monitoring of public policies, will also become an area for development. Policies regarding person-centered care will need to be developed and expanded upon in efforts to support person-centered approaches to quality care in long-term care settings. Although the interpretations of current policies have been expanded to meet the rationale of culture change, more expansion and creative interpretation will be necessary as the long-term care movement strives to work against outcomes of loneliness, hopelessness, and a lack of connection to others.

Finally, efforts to document outcomes through research and evaluation will be paramount as efforts to support a person-centered approach to long-term care is moved forward. Health and human services now exist within a world of "evidence," and evidence-based decision-making in the National Pioneer Network has taken strides to begin to document outcomes that result from benchmarking through the Artifacts of Culture Change Tool; however, their efforts are only in the infancy stages. It would be ideal if all facilities were expected to follow the same process for building a database of evidence that is monitored by state coalitions and summarized at a national level. Single-system case study designs can be developed and implemented to support the impact of a person-centered approach to care management for individual residents as a mechanism to document how a person-centered care approach can have an impact at an individual, or micro, level.

And so, the call is to you. Will you push for strategies that will make a difference in the lives of older people? The challenge lies ahead for each one of us. We are the ambassadors of change. We all have a job to do!

DISCUSSION/REFLECTION QUESTIONS

1. *What do you think are three challenges for the future within long-term care settings?*
2. *How do you feel that you could address these challenges?*
3. *How will you begin your role as an ambassador for the culture change movement? What domains will you address initially, and which do you feel have lesser importance?*
4. *How do you envision your role as a professional who has been exposed to the culture change perspective? Will your role be different from that of your peers who work in long-term care settings who have not been exposed to the culture change perspective and benchmarks? If your role is different, explain how you see it to be different.*

REFERENCE

Schoeneman, K., & Bowman, C. (2006). *Development of the Artifacts of Culture Change Tool: Report of Contract HHSM-500-2005-00076P* (Technical report). Baltimore, MD: Centers for Medicaid & Medicare Services. Retrieved from http://www.artifactsofculturechange.org/Data/Documents/artifacts.pdf

APPENDIX A: RESOURCES FOR COMMUNITY-BASED AGENCIES AND NONPROFIT GROUPS

CULTURE CHANGE ORGANIZATIONAL RESOURCES

CALIFORNIA
California Culture Change Coalition
Contact: Darren Trisel, Vice Chair
Phone: 530-888-6257
www.calculturechange.org

COLORADO
Colorado Culture Change Coalition
303 South Broadway, Suite 200-184
Denver, CO 80209
Phone: 303-868-4311
www.coculturechange.org

CONNECTICUT
Connecticut Culture Change Coalition
E-mail: ctculturechange@hotmail.com
www.connecticutculturechange.com

FLORIDA
Florida Pioneer Network
Contact: Annette Kelly, Chairperson
Phone: 407-514-1815
E-mail: kellyarnp@gmail.com
www.floridapioneernetwork.org

GEORGIA
Culture Change Network of Georgia
Contact: Kim McRae
Phone: 770-841-1546
E-mail: kim@haveagoodlife.com
www.culturechangega.org

ILLINOIS
Illinois Pioneer Coalition
639 York Street
Quincy, IL 62301
Phone: 847-420-2828 or 888-434-0008
E-mail: info@illinoispioneercoalition.org
www.Illinoispioneercoalition.org

INDIANA
Indiana Culture Change Coalition
www.indianaculturechangecoalition.webs.com

IOWA
Iowa Person Directed Care Coalition
Phone: 866-236-1430
www.iowapersondirectedcare.org

KENTUCKY
Kentucky Coalition for Person-Centered Care
www.kcpcc.org

LOUISIANA
L.E.A.D.E.R.
Contact: KaraLe Causey, President
7726 Highway 165
Columbia, LA 71418
Phone: 318-235-5002
Fax: 866-616-5893
E-mail: causey@laleader.org
www.laculturechangecoalition.org/

MICHIGAN
Michigan Alliance for Person-Centered Communities
Cean Eppelheimer, Co-chair: 517-927-1875
E-mail: ceppelheimer@phinational.org
Chris Hennessey, Co-chair: 517-483-5204 (hennesc@lcc.edu)
Heather Picotte, Co-chair: 517-896-5706 (picotte@msu.edu)
www.mapcc.info

MINNESOTA
Minnesota Culture Change Coalition
www.mnculturechange.org

MISSOURI
Missouri Coalition Celebrating Care Continuum Change
200 N. Keene Street, Suite 101
Columbia, MO 65201
www.momc5.com
Chair of Board: Joan Devine, RN
Lutheran Senior Services
Director of Performance Improvement
JDevine@LSSLiving.org
Vice Chair of Board: Julie Ballard, RN
Health Systems, Inc.
Director of Culture Change
jballard@health-systems-inc.org

NEBRASKA
Nebraska Aging Enrichment Coalition
Contact: Tami Scheil, Team Leader, Fairview Manor
Phone: 402-268-2271
E-mail: tscheil@fairviewmanor.org
www.necccoalition.org/

NEW MEXICO
Innovation Network of New Mexico, Inc.
5801 Osuna Road NE, Suite 200
Albuquerque, NM 87109
Phone: 505-998-9758
Fax: 505-998-9899
www.innovationnetworkofnm.org

NORTH CAROLINA
North Carolina Coalition for Long Term Care Enhancement
Contact: Becky Wertz, Secretary (becky.wertz@dhhs.nc.gov)
Phone: (919) 855-4580
www.ltcenhance.com

OHIO
Ohio Person-Centered Care Coalition
Contact: Hilary Stai, PC3 Coordinator, Office of the State Long-Term Care Ombudsman
Phone: 614-466-5002
E-mail: info@centeredcare.org
www.centeredcare.org

OREGON
Making Oregon Vital for Elders
13500 SW Pacific Highway, PMB 511
Tigard, OR 97223
E-mail: info@orculturechange.org
www.orculturechange.org

PENNSYLVANIA
Pennsylvania Culture Change Coalition
126 Allen Drive
Beaver, PA 15009
E-mail:questions@paculturechangecoalition.org
www.paculturechangecoalition.org

RHODE ISLAND
RI Generations
www.rigenerations.com

TENNESSEE
TN Eden Alternative Coalition
www.tneden.org

TEXAS
Texas Culture Change Coalition
P.O. Box 705
San Marcos, TX 78667
Phone: 512-938-1127
Fax: 512-938-1008
E-mail: info@txccc.net
www.txccc.net

WISCONSIN
CARE Wisconsin
1840 N. Prospect Avenue.
Milwaukee, WI 53202
www.carewi.org

Wisconsin Coalition for Person Directed Care
Contact: Wanda Plachecki, Coalition Chair
E-mail: plachecki.wanda@co.la-crosse.wi.us
Lakeview Health Center
902 E. Garland Street
West Salem, WI 54669
Phone: 608-786-1400
www.wisconsinpdc.org

APPENDIX B: WEBSITES FOR CULTURE CHANGE RESOURCES

PIONEER AND CULTURE CHANGE WEBSITES

Culture Change Now/Action Pact
http://actionpact.com/

Eden Alternative
http://www.edenalt.org/
This site provides an overview of the Eden Alternative program, mission statement, values and examples of Eden Alternative facilities. It also provides the reviewer with a wealth of information that helps articulate the Eden Alternative concept.

The Green House Project
http://thegreenhouseproject.org/about-us/mission-vision/
This site provides an overview of The Green House Project as envisioned by Bill Thomas, along with stories and examples that portray the project's concepts and objectives.

Illinois Pioneer Coalition
http://www.illinoispioneercoalition.org
This website provides the reader with materials about the culture change processes that have taken place in Illinois. It provides stories from successful culture change efforts, case study examples, and helpful resources that can promote the culture change process.

Institute for Caregiver Education
http://www.caregivereducation.org/
The Institute for Caregiver Education is a nonprofit organization that provides continuing education and professional development opportunities for health care professionals, including a variety of literacy, language, and life skills training for entry-level staff across all disciplines.

Making Oregon Vital for Seniors
http://orculturechange.org/resources/quick-tips-and-tools
This website provides a series of links and resources which can be helpful to older adults seeking out information about the culture change movement.

The National Consumer Voice for Quality Long-Term Care
http://www.theconsumervoice.org/
This site provides resources to consumers and their families which promote advocacy efforts for quality long-term care settings.

National Long-Term Care Ombudsman Resources
http://www.ltcombudsman.org/
The National Long-Term Care Ombudsman Resource Center provides support, technical assistance, and training to the 53 state long-term care ombudsman programs and their statewide networks of almost 600 regional (local) programs. They also provide resources such as documents, reports, and background materials for ombudspeople and advocates representing individuals in long-term care settings.

National Clearinghouse on the Direct Care Workforce
http://www.directcareclearinghouse.org/a_index.jsp
The National Clearinghouse on the Direct Care Workforce is a national online library for people in search of solutions to the direct-care staffing crisis in long-term care.

Pioneer Network
http://www.pioneernetwork.net/
The Pioneer Network is a center for all stakeholders in the field of aging and long-term care whose focus is on providing home and community for elders. This website provides a wealth of resources, from research reports to practice-based examples of culture change.

Resource Kit to Provide Excellence in Alternatives to Nursing Homes
http://www.kdads.ks.gov/LongTermCare/PEAK/Resourcekit.pdf
This toolkit, developed by the Department of Aging, in Kansas, provides a wonderful array of resources for person-centered care, resident empowerment, staff empowerment, and environmental change.

APPENDIX C: GLOSSARY OF CULTURE CHANGE VOCABULARY

This chart provides an overview of common terms used in long-term care facilities. The left-hand column provides the traditional wording, and the right-hand column provides a revised, person-centered language consistent with a culture change paradigm.

Institutional Lingo	Revised Language
Admit: Allowing a person permission to enter a restricted area.	**Move in:** To become a resident of a home or dwelling.
Allow: To give permission to conduct an action.	**Encourage/welcome:** To inspire or stimulate an action by suggesting approval; to foster good regard about an action.
Ambulate: To relocate oneself from location to location via bipedal transportation.	**Walk:** To travel by foot.
Assignment: A task or objective that is expected to be completed by an individual.	**Residents I am caring for:** A person whose comfort, health, and well-being are the responsibility of the person in question.
Assistant: One who gives aid and support to an individual. Acknowledged as superior.	**Associate:** A partner or colleague.
Behaviors: Actions, especially undesirable ones, such as causing a disturbance or striking out at others. Sometimes described as acting out.	**Communication:** The exchange of information between two or more individuals.

(continued)

Institutional Lingo	Revised Language
Charge Nurse: A licensed medical professional who controls the operations of the staff in a designated area.	**Nurse Leader/Neighborhood Nurse Leader:** A licensed medical professional who provides leadership and guidance to his or her team.
Complainer: An individual recognized for issuing excessive complaints.	**A person with concerns:** A person with a vested interest in an issue or the well-being of an individual.
Confused: Unable to think with clarity.	**Living in the past:** Given to frequent reminiscences of prior experiences.
Control: To restrain through domination or assertion of superiority.	**Facilitate/mentor/influence/guide:** To assist the progress of a person or group through education; to advise or supervise others in order to help the individual or group improve.
Dietary: A term that relates to the biological function of digesting foodstuffs.	**Dining services:** A group of staff members who serve the nutritional needs of residents.
Direct: To give commands to others, backed by an understood or perceived authority.	**Lead/influence:** To guide through example; to impel others to act a certain way.
Discharge: To end a professional or clinical situation, as at the end of a military career or hospital stay; to send away.	**Move out:** To discontinue one's residence in a home or dwelling.
Discipline: Punishment assigned for purposes of correction; used for breaches of an established order or code of conduct.	**Coaching/counseling:** Advice or instruction offered to direct the conduct of others through appeals to the intellect or emotions.
Discipline: A profession that requires specialized training.	**Department:** A division of a business that manages a particular aspect of the company. **Area of expertise:** Special skill or knowledge.
Elope: To vacate the premises without permission or official leave.	**Unescorted exit/left the building:** To leave without notifying those responsible for your care.
Expired: No longer useful or viable, as with spoiled food or drivers' licenses.	**Died:** No longer living or lacking functions necessary to sustain life. **Passed away:** A phrase commonly used to express that someone has died.

APPENDIX C: GLOSSARY OF CULTURE CHANGE VOCABULARY

Institutional Lingo	Revised Language
Facility: A building or compound built to serve a specific function or service, as in educational, medical, military, or transportation facilities.	**Community:** A social group composed of individuals or families who share a common locality and who often share a common culture. **Home:** A place where a person finds comfort and security: "Where the heart is."
Feeder: One who is fed by another; in other contexts, a reference to livestock that is being fattened for the market.	**Person who needs assistance with dining:** A human being who needs someone to contribute to the fulfillment of needs related to eating.
Focus on task: Dedication to completing an assigned duty or piece of work.	**Focus on behavior:** Emphasis on how a person conducts him- or herself.
Front line staff/line staff: Employees who carry out the work of an establishment in direct contact with the customer. Often referred to as those in the most direct "line of fire."	**Care team members/care team associates:** Persons associated with a common goal and whose role is to be attentive and provide assistance or treatment to those in need.
I AM power: Possessing power over others.	**I empower:** Enabling others to take control over their own affairs.
It's too big a change: What we are inclined to say when the change before us seems overwhelming.	**What are some small changes that will help me get to that big change?** A way to manage success!
Loading up: Securing items in a vehicle for transport, as with cattle on a train car.	**Seating residents in the van:** To place or help (the resident) into or onto a seat.
Lobby/day room: Either an entrance corridor in a public building used as a waiting area, or a room at an institution used for group activities.	**Living room/family room:** An area in a person's home used for recreation, entertaining guests, or other social activities.
Make rounds: To perform repetitive tasks while traveling in a predetermined pattern.	**Check on a resident:** To inquire as to the well-being of an individual.
No: The easiest answer when an individual is asked to do something new or unusual.	**Yes:** A response that often requires some creative thinking and that supports putting people before task. A response that may require the individual to "let go" of preconceived notions or routines. Not necessarily the "easy answer."

(continued)

APPENDIX C: GLOSSARY OF CULTURE CHANGE VOCABULARY

Institutional Lingo	Revised Language
Pass meds: To circulate medications; the act of interchanging medicine between two people.	**Help with meds/Give Mr. Kotovsky his medication:** Assisting a person in accomplishing the task of taking medicine.
Patient: A person under medical care or treatment; often one who suffers from an affliction.	**Elder:** A person who has achieved old age and, with it, the respect of others. A person possessing wisdom and knowledge achieved through a lifetime of experiences. **Guest:** The recipient of others' hospitality; often, one who pays for services provided. **Resident:** A person who dwells in a place.
Perform a task: To complete an assigned duty or piece of work.	**Make a difference:** An act that results in a significant change in the status of events.
Problem: An issue that causes difficulty; an impediment to normal function.	**Challenge:** A test of the abilities of an individual or group, often one that is stimulating to those involved. **Opportunity:** A situation that offers a chance for improvement.
Shipped out: To send away, often through professional channels.	**Taken to the emergency room:** Escorted safely to a destination—in this case, a hospital emergency room.
Smith/Room 241/The fractured hip: Impersonal "shorthand" ways to refer to residents, whether by surname, location, or diagnosis.	**Ms. Smith/Linda:** Respectful ways to refer to residents by the names they prefer.
They: Used to refer to management, corporate, another department, another shift, and so on; a group that does not include the individual referring to it.	**We:** Used to refer to our community, our neighborhood team, our organization's team, and so on; a collective group that does include the individual referring to it.
"'Toilet' the resident": "Toilet" is not even listed in the dictionary as a verb!	**Help the resident to the bathroom:** Give assistance in traveling to a restroom or with restroom activities.
To service: To repair or restore to working condition, as with automobiles.	**To provide care for:** To watch over; to serve in a compassionate capacity.
Transport to: To move from one place to another, as with freight.	**Assist:** To support; to render aid in a time of need.

Institutional Lingo	Revised Language
Trying to find who was at fault: Seeking out a person to whom blame can be assigned for a flaw or failing.	**Trying to find the reason it happened:** Searching for the root cause of a problem or mistake.
What's wrong: Determining what is inappropriate or out of order.	**What's right:** Determining what is correct or proper.

Adapted from Devine, J. (2009). *Word of the Week: Building a Culture Change Dictionary*. St. Louis, MO: Lutheran Social Services. With permission.

BIBLIOGRAPHY

Altus, D. E., Engelman, K. K., & Mathews, R. M. (2002). Using family-style meals to increase participation and communication in persons with dementia. *Journal of Gerontological Nursing, 28*(9), 47–53.

Barry, T. (2005). Nurse aide empowerment strategies and staff stability: Effects on nursing home resident outcomes. *The Gerontologist, 45*(3), 309–317.

Bergman-Evans, B. (2004). Beyond the basics: Effects of the Eden Alternative model on quality of life issues. *Journal of Gerontological Nursing, 30*(6), 27–34.

Bishop, C. E., Squillace, M. R., Meagher, J., Anderson, W. L., & Wiener, J. M. (2009). Nursing home work practices and nursing assistants' job satisfaction. *The Gerontologist, 49*(5), 611–622. doi:10.1093/geront/gnp040

Bond, G. E., & Fiedler, F. E. (1999). A comparison of leadership vs. renovation in changing staff values. *Nursing Economics, 17*(1), 37–43.

Borg, M., Karlsson, B., Tondora, J., & Davidson, L. (2009). Implementing person-centered care in psychiatric rehabilitation: What does this involve? *The Israel Journal of Psychiatry and Related Sciences, 46*(2), 84–93.

Brannon, S., Kemper, P., Heier-Leitzell, B., & Stott, A. (2010). Reinventing management practices in long-term care: How cultural evolution can affect workforce recruitment and retention. *Generations, 34*(4), 68–74.

Brune, K. (2011). Culture change in long term care services: Eden-greenhouse-aging in the community. *Educational Gerontology, 37*(6), 506–525. doi:10.1080/03601277.2011.570206

Buettner, L. (2009). Culture change and activities: Learning the lingo and making yourself invaluable. *Activities Directors' Quarterly for Alzheimer's & Other Dementia Patients, 10*(1), 27–32.

Calkins, M., & Casella, C. (2007). Exploring the cost and value of private versus shared bedrooms in nursing homes. *The Gerontologist, 47*(2), 169–183.

Calkins, M., Kator, M., Wyatt, A., & Halliday, L. (2009). Culture change in action: Changing the experiential environment. *Long-Term Living: For the Continuing Care Professional, 58*(11), 16.

Caspar, S., O'Rourke, N., & Gutman, G. M. (2009). The differential influence of culture change models on long-term care staff empowerment and provision of individualized care. *Canadian Journal on Aging, 28*(2), 165–175.

Chapin, M. K. (2010). The language of change: Finding words to define culture change in long-term care. *Journal of Aging, Humanities, and the Arts, 4*(3), 185–199. doi:10.1080/19325614.2010.508332

Clayson, L. (2007). Person-centered care. *Nursing Standard, 21*(49), 59.
Cohen-Mansfield, J., Marx, M. S., Thein, K., & Dakheel-Ali, M. (2010). The impact of past and present preferences on stimulus engagement in nursing home residents with dementia. *Aging and Mental Health, 14*(1), 67–73.
Cohen-Mansfield, J., Parpura-Gill, A., & Golander, H. (2006). Utilization of self-identity roles for designing interventions for persons with dementia. *Journals of Gerontology: Series B: Psychological Sciences and Social Sciences, 61*(4), P202–P212.
Coleman, M. T., Looney, S., O'Brien, J., Ziegler, C., Pastorino, C. A., & Turner, C. (2002). The Eden alternative: Findings after 1 year of implementation. *Journals of Gerontology: Series A: Biological Sciences and Medical Sciences, 57*(7), 422–427.
Crandall, L. G., White, D. L., Schuldheis, S., & Talerico, K. A. (2007). Initiating person-centered care practices in long-term care facilities. *Journal of Gerontological Nursing, 33*(11), 47–56.
Curry, L., Porter, M., Michalski, M., & Gruman, C. (2000). Individualized care: Perceptions of certified nurse's aides. *Journal of Gerontological Nursing, 26*(7), 45–51.
Cutler, L. J., & Kane, R. A. (2009). Post-occupancy evaluation of a transformed nursing home: The first four Green House® settings. *Journal of Housing for the Elderly, 23*(4), 304–334.
Dilley, L., & Geboy, L. (2010). Staff perspectives on person-centered care in practice. *Alzheimer's Care Today, 11*(3), 172–185.
DiLollo, A., & Favreau, C. (2010). Person-centered care and speech and language therapy. *Seminars in Speech & Language, 31*(2), 90–97. doi:10.1055/s-0030-1252110
Dudley-Finnan, S. (2007). Person-centred care. *Nursing Standard, 21*(33), 59.
Edvardsson, D., Fetherstonhaugh, D., McAuliffe, L., Nay, R., & Chenco, C. (2011). Job satisfaction amongst aged care staff: Exploring the influence of person-centered care provision. *International Psychogeriatrics, 23*(8), 1205–1212.
Edvardsson, D., Fetherstonhaugh, D., Nay, R., & Gibson, S. (2010). Development and initial testing of the Person-centered Care Assessment Tool (P-CAT). *International Psychogeriatrics, 22*(1), 101–108.
Edvardsson, D., & Innes, A. (2010). Measuring person-centered care: A critical comparative review of published tools. *The Gerontologist, 50*(6), 834–846.
Ekman, I., Swedberg, K., Taft, C., Lindseth, A., Norberg, A., Brink, E., ... Sunnerhagen, K. S. (2011). Person-centered care—Ready for prime time. *European Journal of Cardiovascular Nursing, 10*, 248–251. doi:10.1016/j.ejcnurse.2011.06.008
Elliot, A. E. (2010). Occupancy and revenue gains from culture change in nursing homes: A win–win innovation for a new age of long-term care. *Seniors Housing & Care Journal, 18*(1), 61–76.
Fagan, R. (2003). Pioneer network: Changing the culture of aging in America. *Journal of Social Work in Long-Term Care, 2*(1/2), 125–140.
Flesner, M. K. (2009). Person-centered care and organizational culture in long-term care. *Journal of Nursing Care Quality, 24*(4), 273–276.
Forbes-Thompson, S., Leiker, T., & Bleich, M. R. (2007). High-performing and low-performing nursing homes: A view from complexity science. *Health Care Management Review, 32*(4), 341–351. doi:10.1097/01.HMR.0000296789.39128.f6

Frandsen, B. (2009). Inspiring a culture change journey. *Long-Term Living: For the Continuing Care Professional, 58*(8), 38–39.
Friedemann, M. L., Montgomery, R. J., Maiberger, B., & Smith, A. A. (1997). Family involvement in the nursing home: Family-oriented practices and staff–family relationships. *Research in Nursing and Health, 20*(6), 527–537.
Geboy, L. (2009a). Linking person-centered care and activity programming. *Alzheimer's Care Today, 10*(3), 156–171.
Geboy, L. (2009b). Linking person-centered care and the physical environment: 10 design principles for elder and dementia care staff. *Alzheimer's Care Today, 10*(4), 228–231.
Gibson, D. E., & Barsade, S. G. (2003). Managing organizational culture change: The case of long-term care. *Journal of Social Work in Long-Term Care, 2*(1/2), 11–34.
Gil, H. (2011). Culture change ideas that work. *Provider, 37*(4), 45. Retrieved from http://www.providermagazine.com/archives/archives-2011/Pages/0411/Culture-Change-Ideas-That-Work.aspx
Gruss, V., McCann, J. J., Edelman, P., & Farran, C. J. (2004). Job stress among nursing home certified nursing assistants: Comparison of empowered and non-empowered work environments. *Alzheimer's Care Today, 5*(3), 207.
Hertzberg, A., & Ekman, S. L. (2000). "We, not them and us?" Views on the relationships and interactions between staff and relatives of older people permanently living in nursing homes. *Journal of Advanced Nursing, 31*(3), 614–622.
Hill, N. L., Kolanowski, A. M., Milone-Nuzzo, P., & Yevchak, A. (2011). Culture change models and resident health outcomes in long-term care. *Journal of Nursing Scholarship, 43*(1), 30–40. doi:10.1111/j.1547-5069.2010.01379.x
Hoeffer, B., Talerico, K. A., Rasin, J., Mitchell, C. M., Stewart, B. J., McKenzie, D., ... Sloane, P. D. (2006). Assisting cognitively impaired nursing home residents with bathing: Effects of two bathing interventions on caregiving. *The Gerontologist, 46*(4), 524–532.
Hughes, R. G. (2011). Overview and summary: Patient-centered care. Challenges and rewards. *Online Journal of Issues in Nursing, 16*(2). doi:10.3912/OJIN. Vol16No02ManOS
Janes, N., Sidani, S., Cott, C., & Rappolt, S. (2008). Figuring it out in the moment: A theory of unregulated care providers' knowledge utilization in dementia care settings. *Worldviews on Evidence-Based Nursing, 5*(1), 13–24.
Jarrott, S. E., & Gigliotti, C. M. (2010). Comparing responses to horticultural-based and traditional activities in dementia care programs. *American Journal of Alzheimer's Disease and Other Dementias, 25*(8), 657–665.
Jones, C. S. (2011). Person-centered care: The heart of culture change. *Journal of Gerontological Nursing, 37*(6), 18–23. doi:10.3928/00989134-20110302-04
Kane, R. A., Lum, T. Y., Cutler, L. J., Degenholtz, H. B., & Yu, T. C. (2007). Resident outcomes in small-house nursing homes: A longitudinal evaluation of the initial Green House® program. *Journal of the American Geriatrics Society, 55*(6), 832–839.
Katz, R. E., & Frank, R. G. (2010–2011). A vision for the future: New care delivery models can play a vital role in building tomorrow's eldercare workforce. *Journal of the American Society of Aging, 34*(4), 82–88.
Kelly, J. (2007). Barriers to achieving patient-centered care in Ireland. *Dimensions of Critical Care Nursing, 26*(1), 29–34.
Kelly, M., & McSweeney, E. (2009). Re-visioning respite: A culture change initiative in a long-term care setting in Eire. *Quality in Ageing, 10*(3), 4–11.

King, S. P., O'Brien, C. J., Edelman, P., & Fazio, S. (2011). Evaluation of the person-centered care essentials program: Importance of trainers in achieving targeted outcomes. *Gerontology & Geriatrics Education, 32*(4), 379–395. doi:10.1080/02701960.2011.611552

Koren, M. J. (2010). Person-centered care for nursing home Residents: The culture-change movement. *Health Affairs, 29*(2), 1–6.

Kostiwa, I., & Meeks, S. (2009). The relation between psychological empowerment, service quality, and job satisfaction among certified nursing assistants. *Clinical Gerontologist, 32*(3), 276–292.

LaPorte, M. (2010). Culture change goes mainstream: Green House homes, considered the pinnacle of the movement, have spread to 26 states. *Provider, 36*(5), 22.

Lawton, M. P., Van Haitsma, K., Klapper, J., Kleban, M. H., Katz, I. R., & Corn, J. (1998). A stimulation–retreat special care unit for elders with dementing illness. *International Psychogeriatrics, 10*(4), 379–395.

Lehning, A., & Austin, M. (2010). Long-term care in the United States: Policy themes and promising practices. *Journal of Gerontological Social Work, 53*(1), 43–63. doi:10.1080/01634370903361979

LeRoy, L., Treanor, K., & Art, E. (2010). Foundation work in long-term care. *Health Affairs, 29*, 207–211. doi:10.1377/hlthaff.2009.0783

Leutz, W., Bishop, C. E., & Dodson, L. (2010). Role for a labor–management partnership in nursing home person-centered care. *The Gerontologist, 50*(3), 340–351.

Lopez, S. (2006). Culture change management in long-term care: A shop-floor view. *Politics & Society, 34*(1), 55–80. doi:10.1177/0032329205284756

Love, K., & Kelly, A. (2011). Person-centered care: changing with the times. *Geriatric Nursing, 32*, 125–129.

Lum, T. Y., Kane, R. A., Cutler, L. J., & Yu, T. C. (2008). Effects of Green House® nursing homes on residents' families. *Health Care Financing Review, 30*(2), 35–51.

Lynch, J. (2009). Leadership in person-centered dementia care. *Nursing Older People 21*(9). Supplement, 11.

Manley, K., & McCormack, B. (2008). Person-centered care. *Nursing Management, 15*(8), 12–13.

Matthews, E. A., Farrell, G. A., & Blackmore, A. M. (1996). Effects of an environmental manipulation emphasizing client-centered care on agitation and sleep in dementia sufferers in a nursing home. *Journal of Advanced Nursing, 24*(3), 439–447.

McFadden, S. H., & Lunsman, M. (2010). Continuity in the midst of change: Behaviors of residents relocated from a nursing home environment to small households. *American Journal of Alzheimer's Disease and Other Dementias, 25*(1), 51–57.

Medvene, L., Grosch, K., & Swink, N. (2006). Interpersonal complexity: A cognitive component of person-centered care. *The Gerontologist, 46*(2), 220–226.

Mezzich, J., Snaedal, J., van Weel, C., & Health, I. (2010). Toward person-centered medicine: From disease to patient to person. *Mount Sinai Journal of Medicine, 77*(3), 304–306. doi:10.1002/msj.20187

Mickus, M. A., Wagenaar, D. B., Averill, M., Colenda, C. C., Gardiner, J., & Luo, Z. (2002). Developing effective bathing strategies for reducing problematic behavior for residents with dementia: The PRIDE approach. *Journal of Mental Health and Aging, 8*, 37–43.

Misiorski, S. (2003). Pioneering culture change. *Nursing Homes: Long Term Care Management, 52*(10), 24–31.
Misiorski, S., & Kahn, K. (2005). Changing the culture of long-term care: Moving beyond programmatic change. *Journal of Social Work in Long-Term Care, 3*(3/4), 137–146.
Moore, K. S. (2005). Review of "Culture Change in Long-Term Care." *Educational Gerontology, 31*(1), 83–85. doi:10.1080/03601270590900107
Norton, E. S. (2010). Sustaining a person-centered care environment. *Long-Term Living: For the Continuing Care Professional, 59*(8), 40–42.
O'Neil, T. (2009). Adding families to the care team: Family members hold keys to person centered care. *Health Progress, 90*(6), 48–50.
Peck, R. L. (2011). Time for change: My top 10 movements in long-term care. *Long-Term Living: For the Continuing Care Professional, 60*(5). Retrieved from http://www.ltlmagazine.com/article/my-top-10-movements-long-term-care
Pfefferle, S., & Weinberg, D. (2008). Certified nurse assistants making meaning of direct care. *Qualitative Health Research, 18*(7), 952–961.
Phillips, L. J., Reid-Arndt, S. A., & Pak, Y. (2010). Effects of a creative expression intervention on emotions, communication, and quality of life in persons with dementia. *Nursing Research, 59*(6), 417.
Pongsupap, Y., & Van Leberghe, W. (2011). People-centered medicine and WHO's renewal of primary health care. *Journal of Evaluation in Clinical Practice, 17*(2), 339–340. doi:10.1111/j.1365-2753.2010.01587.x
Price, B. Exploring person-centered care. (2006). *Nursing Standard, 20*(50), 49–56; quiz, 58.
Ragsdale, V., & McDougall, G. J. (2008). The changing face of long-term care: Looking at the past decade. *Issues in Mental Health Nursing, 29*(9), 992–1001. doi:10.1080/01612840802274818
Rahman, A., Straker, J. K., & Manning, L. (2009). Staff assignment practices in nursing homes: Review of the literature. *Journal of the American Medical Directors Association, 10*(1), 4–10.
Redfoot, D. L. (2003). The changing consumer: The social context of culture change in long-term care. *Journal of Social Work in Long-Term Care, 2*(1/2), 95–110.
Reimer, H. D., & Keller, H. H. (2009). Mealtimes in nursing homes: Striving for person-centered care. *Journal of Nutrition for the Elderly, 28*(4), 327–347.
Remsburg, R. E., Luking, A., Baran, P., Radu, C., Pineda, D., Bennett, R. G., & Tayback, M. (2001). Impact of a buffet-style dining program on weight and biochemical indicators of nutritional status in nursing home residents: A pilot study. *Journal of the American Dietetic Association, 101*(12), 1460–1463.
Robinson, S. B., & Rosher, R. B. (2006). Tangling with the barriers of culture change: Creating a resident-centered nursing home environment. *Journal of Gerontological Nursing, 32*(10), 19–25.
Ronch, J. L. (2011). Organizational approach to preferred view. *Long-Term Living: For the Continuing Care Professional, 60*(3), 16–18.
Rosher, R. B., & Robinson, S. (2005). Impact of the Eden Alternative on family satisfaction. *Journal of the American Medical Directors Association, 6*(3), 189–193.
Scalzi, C. C., Evans, L. K., Barstown, A., & Hostvedt, K. (2006). Barriers and enablers to changing organizational culture in nursing homes. *Nursing Administration Quarterly, 30*(4), 368–372.
Schnelle, J. F., Bertrand, R. Hurd, D., White, A., Squires, D., Feuerberg, M., ... Simmons, S. F. (2009). Resident choice and the survey process: The need for

standardized observation and transparency. *The Gerontologist, 49*(4), 517–524. doi:10.1093/geront/gnp050

Shura, F., Siders, R. A., & Dannefer, D. (2011). Culture change in long-term care: Participatory action research and the role of the resident. *The Gerontologist, 51*(2), 212–225.

Simard, J., & Volicer, L. (2010). Effects of namaste care on residents who do not benefit from usual activities. *American Journal of Alzheimer's Disease and Other Dementias, 25*, 46–51.

Sloane, P. D., Hoeffer, B., Mitchell, C. M., McKenzie, D. A., Barrick, A. L., Rader, J., … Koch, C. G. (2004). Effect of person-centered showering and the towel bath on bathing-associated aggression, agitation, and discomfort in nursing home residents with dementia: A randomized, controlled trial. *Journal of the American Geriatrics Society, 52*(11), 1795–1804.

Slocombe, P. (2003). Using strengths-based practice to support culture change: An Australian experience. *Journal of Social Work in Long-Term Care, 2*(3/4), 307–323.

Svarstad, B. L., Mount, J. K., & Bigelow, W. (2001). Variations in the treatment culture of nursing homes and responses to regulations to reduce drug use. *Psychiatric Services, 52*(5), 666–672.

Talerico, K., Miller, L., Swafford, K., Radar, J., Sloane, P., & Hiatt, S. (2006). Psychosocial approaches to prevent and minimize pain in people with dementia during morning care. *Alzheimer's Care Today, 7*(3), 163–174.

Tellis-Nayak, V. (2007a). Culture change: Its lapses, anomalies and achievements. *Nursing Homes: Long Term Care Management, 56*(5), 22–23.

Tellis-Nayak, V. (2007b). A person-centered workplace: The foundation for person-centered care giving in long-term care. *Journal of the American Medical Director's Association, 8*(1), 46–54.

Temkin-Greener, H., Zheng, N. T., Cai, S., Zhao, H., & Mukamel, D. B. (2010). Nursing home environment and organizational performance: Association with deficiency citations. *Medical Care, 48*(4), 357–364.

Touhy, T. A., Strews, W., & Brown, C. (2005). Expressions of caring as lived by nursing home staff, residents, and families. *International Journal of Human Caring, 9*(3), 31–37.

Tyler, D. A., & Parker, V. A. (2011). Nursing home culture, teamwork, and culture change. *Journal of Research in Nursing, 16*(1), 37–49.

Ursel, K. L., & Aquino-Russell, C. E. (2010). Illuminating person-centered care with Parse's teaching–learning model. *Nursing Science Quarterly, 23*(2), 118–123. doi:10.1177/0894318410362546

Watts, H. (Ed.). (2006). End-of-life care: Bridging disability and aging with person-centered care. *Issues in Law & Medicine, 21*(3), 275–276.

Wetle, T., Shield, R., Teno, J., Miller, S. C., & Welch, L. (2005). Family perspectives on end-of-life care experiences in nursing homes. *The Gerontologist, 45*(5), 642–650.

Wilkerson, D., & MacDonell, C. (2003). Quality oversight and culture change in long-term care. *Journal of Social Work in Long-Term Care, 2*(3/4), 373–395.

Williams, M. M. (2011). Transformative changes to improve dementia care. *PsycCRITIQUES, 56*(12). doi:10.1037/a0022481

Yeatts, D. E., & Cready, C. M. (2007). Consequences of empowered CNA teams in nursing home settings: A longitudinal assessment. *The Gerontologist, 47*(3), 323–339.

INDEX

accommodation of individual needs, 251–253
ACCT. *See* Artifacts of Culture Change Tool
action stage in stages-of-change model, 203
activities of daily living (ADL), 17, 25
activities, workplace practices benchmarks, 174–175
acute care services, 42
ADA. *See* Americans with Disabilities Act
adaptive door handles, environmental benchmarks, 122–123
adaptive sinks, environmental benchmarks, 122
adequate lighting, 255–257
adequate staffing patterns, 181
ADL. *See* activities of daily living
administrators
    average longevity of, 186
    turnover rates for, 188–189
adult day care programs, 43
adult foster care, 40
advance planning, 213–214
advisory board, 243–244
advocacy, 230
advocate role in coalitions, 237
age
    educational attainment of population 55 years and over by, 22–24
    marital status of age 65 and over population, by, 11
    mobility status of population 55 years and over by, 13–14
age breakdown, 4–10
age groups
    age breakdown within, 4–10
    owner-occupied housing across, 18–20
agendas, 240
aging arena, 211
aging culture, 56
aging movements through coalitions, 242
aging parents, 25
air conditioning controls, environmental benchmarks, 126
almshouses, 31
    concept of, 30
    Elizabethan Poor Laws and, 32
Americans with Disabilities Act (ADA), 122, 127, 242
Architectural Barriers Act, 122
aromatherapy to residents, care practice benchmarks, 97–98
Artifacts of Culture Change Tool (ACCT), 66, 143, 169, 194, 264
    for assessment purposes, 197–198
    bathing calls for rooms, benchmark, 129
    benchmark for dining, 90

283

Artifacts of Culture Change Tool
(ACCT) (*cont.*)
  core principles and values of
    culture change in, 67–68
  development, 62
  domains of, 64, 68–72, 195–196
  environment practice within,
    207, 208
  key areas of culture change
    addressed by, 68–72
  leadership benchmarks in, 157
  orientation to, 261
  perspectives regarding, 64–65
  purpose of, 62–63
  scoring overview of domains
    within, 83
  stages-of-change model using,
    202, 203, 205
assessment process
  documenting, 195
  domains of care, 195–196
  on needs assessments, 197–198
  in strengths-based paradigm, 53
  as tool for success, 193–195
assessment to action process, moving
    from
  behavioral change stages,
    201–204
  change process, 205
  creating homelike environment,
    207–208
  encouraging supervision
    practices, 205–206
  responsiveness of care staff and
    CNAs, 206–207
  transformation stages, 204–205
assisted living facilities, 37–38, 183
authoritarian approach to treatment
    and care, 58
average longevity
  of administrator, 186
  of CNA, 184
  of director of nursing, 186
  of LPNs, 184–185
  of RNs/GNs, 185

baby boomers, 5, 263
baked goods, care practice
    benchmarks, 95–96
Balanced Budget Act, 34–35
baseline benchmarks, 63
bathing
  and bathing schedules, 101–102
  rooms, environmental
    benchmarks, 129–131
  and shower schedules, 102–103
bathroom mirrors, environmental
    benchmarks, 120–121
bedrooms, 257–259
bedtimes, care practice benchmarks,
    100–101
behavioral change, stages of,
    201–204
belief system, 25
benchmarks, 66
  care practice. *See* care practice
    benchmarks
  community. *See* community,
    benchmarks
  environment. *See* environmental
    benchmarks
  for practice in long-term care
    settings, 249
  score
    in care practice, 206, 207
    changes in, 203
  workplace practices. *See*
    workplace practices,
    benchmarks
birthday celebration, care practice
    benchmarks, 96–97
birth rates, after World War II, 5
board-and-care homes, 40
Boren Amendment, 34
Boston's Home for Aged Women, 30
brainstorm alternatives, in
    transformation process,
    204, 205
broader community, 165
Brookhaven Center, 149
buddy systems, 164

buffet style dining option for residents, 91–92

call systems. *See* resident call system
care conferences
    care meetings and, 165–166
    resident, 162–163
career ladders, workplace practices benchmarks, 176
caregivers, 88
    consistency of, 172
care meetings, leadership practice benchmarks, 165–166
care practice benchmarks
    aromatherapy to residents by staff/volunteers, 97–98
    baked goods, 95–96
    bathing
        and bathing schedules, 101–102
        and shower schedules, 102–103
    birthday celebrations, 96–97
    dining. *See* dining styles for residents
    facility pets, 99
    massage to residents by staff/volunteers, 98
    memorials, 105
    person-first care plans, 105–106
    resident pets, 100
    snacks/light refreshments, 95
    support people during their last journey in life, 103–104
care practices
    dignity of individual, 250
    domain, 71
    person-centered care. *See* person-centered care
care providers
    participation between resident and, 231
    team, roles among, 174
care staff, 214
    cross-trained, 207
    responsiveness of, 206–207

care team, supporting, 207
census rates, 189
certified nursing assistant (CNA), 42, 160, 162, 173
    average longevity of, 184
    career ladder positions for, 176
    levels of, 181
    responsiveness of, 206–207
    staff coverage, 189
    turnover rates for, 186–187
    workplace practices benchmarks, 171–172
chairs in public areas, 126–127
"challenging the process" concept, 159–161
change agents, empowerment cultivated by, 212
change culture, effective components of, 62
change process, 64
    behavioral and philosophical changes, 202
    initial steps in, 205
checklist for coalition
    establishing, 243–244
    evaluating effectiveness, 245–246
child day care model, 149
children, family/social support domain, 216
chronic health conditions, 25
cleanliness of areas, issues of, 255
closets, 136
    environmental benchmarks, 123–124
    space, 258
CNA. *See* certified nursing assistant
Coalition of Disability Rights Organizations, 242
coalitions
    building, 233–234
    checklist for establishing and fostering, 243–246
    components of, 234
        agendas, 240

coalitions (*cont.*)
 group roles and responsibilities, 237–239
 key stakeholders, 236–237
 mission statement, 240
 sustainability, 240–242
 vision, 240
 disability and aging movements through, 242
 dynamics of groups and, 235–236
 goal of, 234
 periodic evaluation of, 244
 Pioneer Network and, 242–243
comfortable lighting, 255–256
communication
 building contact list for, 243
 between groups, 234
community
 approach, 58
 benchmarks
  dining areas, 152–154
  food/entertainment provisions, 151–152
  guest rooms, 150–151
  intergenerational relationships, 148–149
  kitchen facilities, 154
  meeting space, 149–150
 engagement, 143–145
 home-based, 12
 meetings, 165
community care settings, 32
community practice
 family and, 143
 settings, implications for, 20–25
companionship, loving, 55
comparative needs, 198
congregate care, 39
consultant role in coalitions, 238
consumer interviews, tools based on, 63
consumer participation, 211–213
 family and, 163, 231
consumer voice, 213
contemplation stage in stages-of-change model, 202–203
continuing-care retirement facilities, 38–39
continuing education, workplace practices benchmarks, 173
contributor role in coalitions, 238
cooking club for residents, 93–94
core values, measured in ACCT, 67–68
critical leadership component, 160
cross-training, workplace practices benchmarks, 174
cultivating relationships, 241
culture change, 25–26
 concept, 34, 195
 environment, 230
 learning circles for, 165
 literature on, 162
 movement, 36, 64, 212
 organizational resources, 265–268
 paradigm, 56–58, 63, 158, 161, 261
  embracing, 66
  future directions, 262–264
  values and principles of, 47
 philosophy, 170
 process, concrete artifacts of, 63
 websites, 269–270
Culture Change Leadership Team, 199
culture of aging, 56
culture of program, 194
current occupancy rate, 189
custodial care, 42

data collection instrument, 62, 65
day care, workplace practices benchmarks, 177
day-to-day challenges to staff, 176
decision-making process, 165, 207
Dekalb (IL) County Rehabilitation and Nursing Center, 92
demand for services. *See* expressed needs
de-medicalization of disability, 52
dietary challenges to staff, 176
dignity of individual, 250
dimming switches in resident rooms, 256

dining areas, community
    benchmarks, 152–154
dining experience, ACCT, 70
dining styles for residents, 90–91
    buffet style, 91–94
    cooking club, 93–94
    family-style approach, 92
    open-dining approach, 92
    restaurant-style, 91
    24-hour dining, 93
director of nursing
    average longevity of, 186
    turnover rates for, 188
disability, 16
    advances in, 242
    arena, 211
    care for people with, 29–30
    de-medicalization of, 52
    movement, 212
    social aspects of, 51
distracters, 235
divorce, older adults, 10
documentation, assessment
    process, 195
dynamics of groups and coalitions,
    235–236

Eden Alternative approach, 35
Eden Alternative experience, 172
Eden Alternative movement, 25
Eden Alternative paradigm,
    55–56
Eden philosophy, guiding principles
    for, 55
educational attainment
    of population 55 years and over,
        22–24
    U.S. Census on, 20
effective care plans, assessment, 196
effective coalitions
    building, 234
    checklist for evaluating,
        245–246
effective leadership, 159
elder-centered community, 55
elderly individuals

culture of treatment and care
    for, 30
poor farms for, 31
Elizabethan Poor Laws, 30, 32
emergency paging, environmental
    benchmarks, 135
employee evaluations, workplace
    practices benchmarks, 178
employee satisfaction, 169
employee turnover, 169
empowerment, 30
    concept of, 212
    process, recovery and, 53
"enabling others to act," leadership
    practice of, 159–161
encourager role in coalitions, 239
"encouraging the heart," 159, 161
end-of-life care in long-term care
    settings, 183
energizer role in coalitions, 238
entertainment provisions, community
    benchmarks, 151–152
entranceways, examples of,
    137–139
environment, 25
    ACCT, 69
    adequate and comfortable
        lighting, 255–257
    elimination of, 254
    homelike, 253–254
    issues of safety and cleanliness, 255
    maintaining, 250
    task-centered, 235
    and well-being, 113
environmental barriers, 54
environmental behavior, 112
environmental benchmarks
    adaptive door handles, 122–123
    adaptive sinks, 122, 123
    bathing rooms, 129–131
    bathroom mirrors, 120–121
    chairs and sofas in public areas,
        126–127
    closets, 123–124
    emergency paging, 135
    gift shop, 128

environmental benchmarks (*cont.*)
  gliders, 127
  heat/air conditioning controls, 126
  internet/computer access, 128–129
  laundry, 135
  lighting, 125
  outdoor garden/patio, 132–133
  outdoor raised gardens, 133–134
  outdoor walking/wheeling path, 134
  pager/radio/call system, 134–135
  privacy-enhanced rooms, 116–118
  private rooms, 116, 117
  refrigerators, 126
  room décor, 124–125
  self-contained household units, 114–116
  towels for resident bathing, 131–132
  traditional nurses' stations, 118–119
  wheelchair-accessible sinks, 121–123
  windows, 120
  workout room, 129, 130
environmental practices, 111–112
evidence-based decision-making, in National Pioneer Network, 263–264
examination of leadership, 157
expert–consumer model, 52
explorations of leadership, 157
expressed needs, 198

facilitate treatment strategies, 49
facility administrators, assessment process for, 194
facility pets, care practice benchmarks, 99
family, 211
  and community benchmarks. *See* community, benchmarks
  engagement, importance of, 143–145
  practices, 143
  and consumer participation, 163, 231
  personal preference inventory components, 215–217
  in planning process, residents and, 213
family collaboration, leadership practice benchmarks, 163–164
family members
  coaching and mentoring of, 163
  elderly, 85
  end-of-life experience for, 183
  guest rooms for, 150–151
  and resident, 105, 133, 222, 241
family-style approach, dining option for residents, 92
fantasy-oriented environments, 263
federal regulatory bodies, 249
felt needs, 197
field of nursing, 48
field of psychiatry, 48
follower role in coalitions, 239
follow-up phase in stages-of-change model, 203
food provisions, community benchmarks, 151–152
foster care units, 173
fostering relationships, 144
functional disability, 145
furniture arrangement, 252–253

gatekeeper role in coalitions, 239
gender
  differences, 10–11
  educational attainment of population 55 years and over by, 22–24
  gap, 10
  marital status of age 65 and over population, by, 11

mobility status of population 55 years and over by, 13–14
65 years and older by, 4–10
general nurses (GNs), average longevity of, 185
germ theory of disease, development of, 49
gift shop for residents, environmental benchmarks, 128
gliders for residents, environmental benchmarks, 127
GNs. *See* general nurses
grandchildren, family/social support domain, 216
Green House Model, 35
group agenda, 240
group homes, 39
    residential care facility versus, 40
group meetings in long-term care facility, 150
group observer role in coalitions, 239
group-oriented members, 235
group roles and responsibilities, 237–239
guest rooms, community benchmarks, 150–151

hallways, renovation of, 136–137
happy hour concept, 144–145
harmonizer role in coalitions, 239
health care system, 32
health/long-term care settings, 47
health status, 16
    racial differences in, 15
    heat conditioning controls, environmental benchmarks, 126
home-based communities, 12
home-based gift shop, 128
home-care services, 42
homelike environment, 253–254
    creation of, 207–208
homes for older adults, 30
hospice care program, 43

Hospital Survey and Reconstruction Act of 1946, 32
household models, 114, 115
    with full kitchen facilities, 154
housekeeping staffs, 175
housing
    designed for seniors, 37
    for individuals who need assistance, 39
    options to older adults, 10
    for people 55+, 15, 18
    tenure, 18–20
        by family type and age of householder 55 years and over, 19
        by household type and age of householder 55 years and over, 21
human dignity, culture of, 66
human services, 47

IADL. *See* instrumental activities of daily living
"I"-format care plans, 105–106
independent living, 37
    options
        assisted living, 37–38
        continuing-care retirement facilities, 38–39
        independent living, 37
        naturally occurring retirement communities, 38
        village concept, 38
    paradigm, 52–53
individual agenda, 240
individualized care
    caregivers, 88
    importance of, 26
    plans, 88, 106
individual needs, accommodation of, 251–253
informational sessions, community meetings, 165
information seeker role in coalitions, 238

inherent strengths, use of, 53
in-home services, 38–39
initiator role in coalitions, 238
in-service program, 144
"inspiring a shared vision," 159, 160, 162
instrumental activities of daily living (IADL), 17, 25
intellectual domain, personal preference inventory components, 220
interests, coalition of, 236–237
intergenerational relationships, community benchmarks, 148–149
intermediate care
　concepts of, 36
　facilities, 33, 34
　for people advancing in age/disabilities, 41
International Classification of Functioning, Disability and Health, 51
internet/computer access, environmental benchmarks, 128–129
interpersonal relationships between residents and staff, 25
interpretive guidelines for residential care. *See* residential care, interpretive guidelines for
involuntary treatment, 50

job development program, workplace practices benchmarks, 176–177

key stakeholders, 236–237
kitchen facilities, community benchmarks, 154

laundry, environmental benchmarks, 135

leadership, 64
　defining, 157–159
　practices, 157, 162
　　benchmarks, 162–166
　　and person-centered care, 160–161
　servant, 158
　structure, 230
　team, 203, 205, 206
　wise, 55
Leadership Practices Inventory, 158
learned helplessness, 112
learning circles, leadership practice benchmarks, 164–165
licensed practical nurses (LPNs), 42
　average longevity of, 184–185
　turnover rates for, 187
　workplace practices benchmarks, 171
Life Safety Code, 257
lighting
　adequate and comfortable, 255–257
　environmental benchmarks, 125
living environment, transformation of, 58
longevity of staff, 184–186
long-term care facilitation, assessment process for, 193–195
long-term care facilities, 87
　create community and social connections in, 147
　dignity and autonomy of elderly people, 261
　from medical model, transformation of, 68
　older adults living in, 132
　opportunities for hospice care in, 137
　residents' voice in, 230
long-term care, implications for, 12, 20–25
long-term care population
　and community practice settings, 20, 25

culture change, 25–26
demographic shift in
    age breakdown, 4–10
    education, 20, 22–24
    health status, 15–17
    housing tenure, 18–20
    marital status, 10–12
    mobility status, 12–14
long-term care settings, 158
    admissions to, 214
    end-of-life care in, 183
    evolution, 29–36
    facilities and, 101
    independent living options. *See* independent living, options
    nursing home care options. *See* nursing home care options
    older adults in, 146
    physical environment plays in lives of residents in, 113
    process of measuring outcomes in, 61
    professionals in, 62–63
    supportive/shelter care options. *See* supportive/shelter care options
    typical day in, 101
LPNs. *See* licensed practical nurses

Main Street Café, 151
maintenance phase in stages-of-change model, 203
management practices, 207
management theories, 157
marital status, 10–12
marriage/long-term relationships, 216
massage to residents, care practice benchmarks, 98
Medicaid programs, 33
    for long-term care, 18
Medical Facilities Survey and Construction Act of 1954, 32
medicalized approach to provision of care, 44
medical model
    approach in nursing home settings, 35
    paradigm, 48–51, 55, 56, 163, 214
    transformation of long-term care facility from, 68
medical nursing services, 24-hour, 41
medical treatment, 55
Medicare, 43, 51, 61
    benefits, 17
    coverage, 33
    programs, 33
meeting space, community benchmarks, 149–150
membership, coalition, 237–239
memorials, care practice benchmarks, 105
mental health arena, 212
mental illness, 30
    behaviors, 48
    problem of, 50
mental vitality, 221–222
Miller Amendment, 33
mission statement, 240
mobility
    status, 12–14
    in terms of ADL and IADL, 25
"modeling the way," 158, 159, 162
    leadership practice of, 160
modern scientific medicine, 49
Moss Amendments, 33
multilevel care facilities, 39

National Center for Health Statistics, 15
nationally prominent facilities, 62
National Pioneer Network, evidence-based decision-making in, 263–264
National Technical Information Service, 254
naturally occurring retirement communities, 38

needs assessments, 197–198
negotiator role in coalitions, 237
New Deal, 31
nonmanagerial staff, standard of paying expenses for, 173
"normalization" concept, 26
normative needs, 197
nursing care, 48
    settings, 29
    skilled, 30
nursing home care options
    acute care services, 42
    adult day care programs, 43
    custodial care, 42
    hospice care program, 43
    intermediate care, 41
    respite care, 43–44
    skilled nursing, 41–42
    subacute care, 42
Nursing Home Reform Act, 34
nursing homes, 25
    ombudsman programs, 34
    quality standards for, 34
    residents, 34
    series of, 170
nursing staff
    activities by, 175
    workplace practice benchmarks, 170–172

occupancy rate, residents, 189
Old Age Assistance (OAA) payments, 31, 32
old-age homes, private, 31
older adults
    care of, 3
    divorce, 10
    health status, 15–17
    homes for, 30
    housing options to, 10
    importance of, 212
    nursing care for, 32
    nursing home, 40–41
    poor farms, 31
    population, 4–5, 35
    research on, 61
    residential and care settings for, 29
ombudsman program, 213
Omnibus Reconciliation Act, 34, 87
on-site day care approach, 149
open-dining approach, dining option for residents, 92
opinion seeker role in coalitions, 238
organizer role in coalitions, 238
outcome practices, 182–183
    benchmarks
        census rates, 189
        longevity of staff, 184–186
        staff coverage, 189
        turnover rates, 186–189
    importance of, 182
    person-centered care, 181–182
outdoor garden/patio, environmental benchmarks, 132–133
outdoor raised gardens, environmental benchmarks, 133–134
outdoor walking/wheeling path, environmental benchmarks, 134
owner-occupied housing, 18, 20

pager, environmental benchmarks, 134–135
participation, self-determination and, 251
patients
    disease condition of, 50
    hospice care, 43
    living in long-term care setting, 99
    organizational assessment, 196
    physician relations to, 50
PCC. *See* person-centered care
people with disabilities, 3
    ADA, 242
    care and treatment of, 32
    intermediate care, 41

long-term care settings, 36
poor farms for, 31
periodic evaluation of coalition, 244
personality attributes, 214
personal preference inventory (PPI)
building, 214–215
case study, 226–230
components of
family/social support, 215–217
intellectual domain, 220
physical/well-being domain, 221–222
recreational domain, 218–220
spirituality domain, 220–221
vocational/occupational domain, 217–218
guide, 222–225
person-centered approach, 35, 44, 56, 208, 212
in long-term care practice, 61
person-centered care (PCC), 181–183, 203
benchmarks, 158
concept of, 25, 87–88
definition, 88
leadership practices and, 160–161
link among, 89–90
model for, 4, 88
philosophy, 170
policies, 263
quality of life and, 35
workplace practices and, 169–170
person-centered environments, 25, 170
person-centered planning, 230
person-first care plans, 105–106
person first needs, 251–253
"person-first" philosophy, 57
Philadelphia's Indigent Widows' and Single Women's Society, 30–31
philosophical paradigm, 47
photovoice method, 212
physically disabled, skilled nursing care to, 30

physical domain, PPI components, 221–222
physicians
for advice and guidance, 50
licensed, 40
medical model approach, 48–49
Pioneering network, 234, 240
pioneer coalitions, 66, 234, 242–243
pioneer movement, 212
Pioneer Network, 149, 242–243, 270
ACCT, 196
benchmark survey, 129, 132
culture change movement, 36
environments and residential alternatives, creation of, 56
process of building culture change paradigm, 67
report published by, 149, 154, 163, 172
pioneers in long-term care, 35
planning process, residents and families in, 213
pneumococcal vaccination, 16
political coalitions, 234
poor farms, people with disabilities, 31
population
55 years and over, educational attainment of, 22–24
older adults in United States, 4
65 years and older, age breakdown within age groups, 4–10
positive well-being care, 89–90
potential outcomes, ACCT, 72
PPI. *See* personal preference inventory
precontemplation stage in stages-of-change model, 202
preparation phase in stages-of-change model, 203
principle-centered approach, 56
privacy-enhanced rooms, environmental benchmarks, 116–117
private old-age homes, 31

private rooms
  environmental benchmarks, 116, 117
  versus shared and greater levels of autonomy, 464
proactive relationships with surveyors, 208
problem solving tool, 165
process of care, 183
process-oriented members, 235, 239
proper diagnosis, 49
Providence Mt. St. Vincent, 151
provision of care, medicalized approach to, 44
psychiatric conditions, 48
psychiatric diagnosis, 53
psychological environment, characteristics of, 113
psychometric properties, ACCT, 63–64

quality of care
  for nursing home residents, 183
  nursing workforce and, 183
quality of life, 15, 183
  and person-centered care, 35
quality of nursing care, 182

racial differences in health status, 15
radio call system, environmental benchmarks, 134–135
realities within medical model, 50
recognition
  in coalition, 241
  to staff, workplace practices benchmarks, 175–176
recovery and empowerment process, 53
recreational domain, personal preference inventory components, 218–220
refrigerators, environmental benchmarks, 126

registered nurses (RNs), 41, 42
  average longevity of, 185
  turnover rates for, 187–188
  workplace practices benchmarks, 170–171
rehabilitation centers/programs in long-term care settings, 51
rehabilitation/disability paradigm, 51–52
rehabilitation services, 42
rehabilitative care, concepts of, 36
relationship building, ACCT, 71
resident call system, 134–135, 259
resident care conferences, leadership practice benchmarks, 162–163
resident choices, ACCT, 70
resident council meetings, 230
residential and care settings for older adults, 29
residential care facilities, 39–40
  versus group home, 40
residential care, interpretive guidelines for
  accommodation of individual needs, 252
  adequate lighting, 256
  dignity of individual, 250
  homelike environment, 253–254
  resident call system, 259
  resident rooms, 257–259
resident pets, care practice benchmarks, 100
residents, 172, 230
  access to computers/internet, 128–129
  adaptive/easy-to-use lever, 122, 123
  adaptive handles, doors, 122–123
  aromatherapy to, 97–98
  avoid labeling clothing, 115
  baked goods within, 96
  bathing rooms, 129–131
  bathroom mirrors, wheelchair accessible and adjustable, 120–122

bath/shower, 102–103
birthday celebration, 96–97
and care providers, 231
CNAs working with, 171
coaching and mentoring of, 163
dining areas, 152–154
dining styles for
  buffet style dining, 91–92
  cooking club, 94
  family-style approach, 92
  food planning options, 91
  open-dining approach for, 92
  restaurant-style dining option, 91
  24-hour dining, 93–94
enabling personal access to refrigerator, 126
facility to keep pets, 99–100
and families in planning process, 213
food/entertainment provisions, 151–152
intergenerational program, children interact with, 148
interpersonal skills, staff and, 88–89
kitchen facilities, 154
massage to, 98
meaningful and long-lasting relationships with, 170
meeting space, 149–150
memorials/remembrances for individual, 105
nurses working with, 170–171
outdoor garden/patio, 132–133
outdoor raised gardens available for, 133–134
pager/radio/telephone call system, calls register from, 134–135
PCC focused on, 87
personal clothing, 135
physical environment, 252–253
in PPI, family members and, 222
principles, 57

in privacy-enhanced shared rooms, 116–118
with private dining rooms, 152–153
in private rooms, 116
relationship building between staff and, 71
rights, 57
room, 257–259
  adjustable air conditioning controls in, 126
  dimming switches in, 256
  example of personalizing, 124
  floor lamps and reading lamps in, 125
smaller community of, 114
snacks/drinks, availability for, 95
and staff, 144
store/gift shop/cart available for purchase, 128
waking times/bedtimes chosen by, 100–101
warm towels for bathing, 131–132
windows facilities in, 120
workout room available to, 129, 130
resources
  culture change organizational, 265–268
  stakeholder, 236–237
respite care, 43–44
restaurant-style dining option for residents, 91
retirement communities, 37, 150
rewards for members, 242
RNs. *See* registered nurses
room décor, environmental benchmarks, 124–125

same-sex relationships, 262–263
scheduling, workplace practices benchmarks, 172–173

scrubs. *See* uniforms, workplace practices benchmarks
self-advocacy movement, 211
self-assessment, ACCT, 71
self-contained household units, environmental benchmarks, 114–116
self-determination and participation, 251
servant leadership, 158
service delivery arena, 212
service network's governance process, 212
setting for care, 44
shared vision, concept of inspiring, 159
Shell Point Retirement Community in Fort Meyers, 150
shelter
　care options. *See* Supportive/shelter care options
　elderly individuals need of, 30
short-term rehabilitation, 42
shower schedules, bathing and, 102–103
siblings, family/social support domain, 216
skilled nursing, 33, 41–42
　care to physically disabled, 30
smoking behaviors in culture change, 202
snacks/light refreshments to residents, care practice benchmarks, 95
social environment, 52, 113
social isolation, 146
Social Security Act of 1935, 31
Social Security program, 32
　Amendments to, 33
social support, 43, 145
　family/social support domain, 216–217
　personal preference inventory components, 215–217
　and well-being, 145–48

sofas in public areas, 126–127
special homes to care for elderly people, 30
spirituality domain, personal preference inventory components, 220–221
spokesperson role in coalitions, 237
staff, 158
　activities, informal/formal by, 175
　within care practices of residents, 162–163
　consistent assignment of, 172
　coverage, 189
　cross-training for, 174
　day care by, 177
　empowerment, ACCT, 70–71
　job development program to, 176–177
　positions, 170
　recognition to, 175–176
　and residents, 71
　roles of, 171, 212
　shortages of, 172
　uniforms/scrubs, 173–174
staffing outcomes, 182
stages-of-change model, 202–204, 208
stakeholders, 236
　groups, 63
　impact for, 63
　levels of, 160
standard setter role in coalitions, 239
standards of care, 33
standards of excellence, 158
state regulatory bodies, 249
sterile institutional approach to community approach, 58
strengths-based approach, 53, 54
strengths-based paradigm, 53–54
　principles for, 54
subacute care, 42
　concepts of, 34, 36
substance use and access, 262
Sunny Home Nursing Center of Joliet, 149

supervision practices
  building, 207
  encouraging new models of, 205–206
supportive/shelter care options
  adult foster care, 40
  board-and-care homes, 40
  congregate care, 39
  group homes, 39
  residential care facilities, 39–40
surveyors, proactive relationships with, 208
sustainability, coalition component, 240–242

task-centered environment, 235
task-oriented members, 235, 239
technological lifestyle, 263
Teresian House, 151
test–retest reliability, 63
Texas Long Term Care Institute, 56
therapist, power and authority barrier between person and, 54
"Through the Looking Glass," 175
tool for success, assessment as, 193–195
top-down bureaucratic authority, de-emphasizing, 55
towels for resident bathing, environmental benchmarks, 131–132
traditional culture of care, 56–57
traditional nursing stations
  elimination of, 69
  environmental benchmarks, 118–119
traditional public announcement system, 69
transformation
  stages of, 204–205
  of working/living environment, 58
transformational leadership strategies, 158–159

transformative efforts, domains in, 36
turnover rates
  for administrators, 188–189
  for CNA, 186–187
  for directors of nursing, 188
  for LPNs, 187
  for RNs, 187–188
24-hour dining option for residents, 93
24-hour nursing care, 41

uniforms, workplace practices benchmarks, 173–174
U.S. Census Bureau, 4, 20

"victim identity," 53
village concept, 38
vision, 64
  component of coalition, 240
visitors, guest rooms for, 150
vocational/occupational domain, personal preference inventory components, 217–218
volunteers, 164
  coordinator, workplace practices benchmarks, 177

well-being care, positive, 89–90
well-being domain, PPI components, 221
wheelchair-accessible sinks, environmental benchmarks, 121–123
wheelchair-bound residents, 154
windows, environmental benchmarks, 120
wireless systems, 259
women, age group, 10
working environment, transformation of, 58
working with coalitions, 236

workout room to residents,
    environmental benchmarks,
    129, 130
workplace practices
    benchmarks
        activities, 174–175
        career ladders, 176
        CNAs, 171–172
        continuing education, 173
        cross-training, 174
        day care, 177
        employee evaluations, 178
        job development, 176–177
        licensed practical nurses, 171
        recognition, 175–176
        registered nurses, 170–171
        scheduling, 172–173
        uniforms, 173–174
        volunteer coordinator, 177
    and person-centered care, 169–170
World Health Organization, 51